THE
EMOTIONAL
ROOTS
OF
CHRONIC ILLNESS

"Enlightening, erudite, engaging, and expressive. I like the local links between the five senses, the five Chinese phases, and the five main miasms. The remedy portraits are picturesque, with delicately descriptive themes, sublime application of astute language, all in a context of world literature, philology, and religion. Kantor's use of language is masterful and highly engaging. I truly enjoyed reading it."

FRANS VERMEULEN, AUTHOR, LECTURER, AND
AUTHORITY ON MATERIA MEDICA

"This remarkable synthesis of cutting-edge knowledge is rooted in ancient practices of Traditional Chinese Medicine as well as in homeopathy's futuristic, Western medical tradition. Five revelatory existential questions are introduced. Convincingly, each provides the subtext for health, epigenetics, and emergent chronic illness. Offering case histories, clinical pearls, Greek myth analysis, and much more, Kantor's book is a stunning yet enjoyable read. Highly recommended."

DANA ULLMAN, MPH, CCH,
AUTHOR OF *THE HOMEOPATHIC REVOLUTION*

"This book by Jerry Kantor gives good insights in the reactions between medicine and psychology. It points to the source of disease as psychological. Added to that is its relationship with philosophy, which gives his work even further depth. It is a great book."

JAN SCHOLTEN, M.D.,
AUTHOR OF *HOMEOPATHY AND THE ELEMENTS*

"Jerry Kantor is a gifted and experienced homeopath who thinks deeply about homeopathy and its applications to living beings. He has written this well-thought-out, highly philosophical book that gets the reader to think about one's existential reality and roots, to learn more about homeopathy, and see how both relate to Traditional Chinese Medicine. He makes some easy-to-understand analogies using familiar movie and literary characters to make his points easier to understand. An incredibly intellectual and poignant read!"

ABBY BEALE, RSHOM (NA), CERTIFIED CLASSICAL HOMEOPATH

"A tour de force of the philosophical and existential themes inherent in a homeopathic understanding of illness, Kantor provides a newly emerging synthesis of the relationship between miasmatic human conditions and the life-enhancing force of nature's own substances encased within homeopathic remedies."

LORETTA BUTEHORN, PH.D., CERTIFIED
CLASSICAL HOMEOPATH AND PSYCHOLOGIST

"This well-researched synthesis of many classical healing systems with historical references focuses on homeopathy. The first section is an introduction to homeopathy and a very useful, in-depth description of the homeopathic healing process. The section of miasms and the Five Elements of Traditional Chinese Medicine is particularly interesting. Kantor delves into historical and medical insights that flesh out Hahnemann's original theory of miasms."

JANE TARA CICCHETTI, AUTHOR OF
DREAMS, SYMBOLS, AND HOMEOPATHY

"Kantor provides an insightful overview of five core existential dilemmas that life presents, positing that our responses to these quandaries become embodied in specific symptoms and syndromes of mind and body. His breathtaking perspective on the human condition will amply reward readers, from the lay public to professionals of any medical persuasion."

DAVID C. KAILIN, MPH, PH.D.,
AUTHOR OF QUALITY IN COMPLEMENTARY & ALTERNATIVE MEDICINE

"Kantor uses his exceptional mastery of wit, metaphor, and integrative healing resources to help us understand how unique emotional and physical symptoms emerge as guides to mend the manifestations of chronic illness."

KENNETH SILVESTRI, ED.D., CERTIFIED
HOMEOPATH AND PSYCHOTHERAPIST

"Are you familiar with the sufferings (or inner torments) of the mythical Greek god Sisyphus, Hamlet Prince of Denmark, Bartelby the Scrivener, and Phil Connors of the movie *Groundhog Day*? Jerry Kantor's analysis of their existential plights and the remedy each needs is worth the price of admission."

ANURADHA DAYAL-GULATI, PH.D., AUTHOR OF
HEAL YOUR ANCESTRAL ROOTS

"Insightful and thought-provoking. The first book to bring together existential philosophy, miasms, and homeopathic solutions! Gripping in content and lucid in style. We enjoyed reading the book and so will every reader!"

DR. BHAWISHA & DR. SHACHINDRA JOSHI, M.D. (HOM),
MUMBAI, INDIA

THE
EMOTIONAL
ROOTS
OF
CHRONIC
ILLNESS

Homeopathy
for Existential Stress

JERRY M. KANTOR

Healing Arts Press
Rochester, Vermont

Healing Arts Press
One Park Street
Rochester, Vermont 05767
www.HealingArtsPress.com

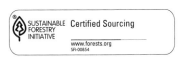

Text stock is SFI certified

Healing Arts Press is a division of Inner Traditions International

Copyright © 2023 by Jerry M. Kantor

All rights reserved. No part of this book may be reproduced or utilized in any form or by any means, electronic or mechanical, including photocopying, recording, or by any information storage and retrieval system, without permission in writing from the publisher.

Note to the reader: *This book is intended as an informational guide. The remedies, approaches, and techniques described herein are meant to supplement, and not to be a substitute for, professional medical care or treatment. They should not be used to treat a serious ailment without prior consultation with a qualified health care professional.*

Cataloging-in-Publication Data for this title is available from the Library of Congress

ISBN 978-1-64411-784-2 (print)
ISBN 978-1-64411-785-9 (ebook)

Printed and bound in the United States by Lake Book Manufacturing, LLC
The text stock is SFI certified. The Sustainable Forestry Initiative® program promotes sustainable forest management.

10   9   8   7   6   5   4   3   2   1

Text design and layout by Virginia Scott Bowman
This book was typeset in Garamond Premier Pro, Frutiger, and Gill Sans with Raleway used as the display typeface

To send correspondence to the author of this book, mail a first-class letter to the author c/o Inner Traditions • Bear & Company, One Park Street, Rochester, VT 05767, and we will forward the communication, or contact the author directly at **vitalforcehealthcare.com**.

✦ ✦

To the memory of Mary Cheevers McKenzie

Contents

PART ONE
A Homeopathic Framework

PART TWO
Five Existential Questions
And Their Corresponding Miasms,
Sense Dimensions, Phases, Emotions, and Organs

Foreword

As teenagers roaming the pine woods in search of wildflowers, my best friend and I pursued a deeper quest as well, pondering what we called "the great questions of Life, Death, God, and the Universe." Or lying on our backs in a field of sweet timothy grass, we would watch the white puffy clouds sail by and wonder . . . *Who am I, and what am I doing here? . . . Does God exist? . . . What happens after we die?* Searching for answers, we read *Siddhartha, The Teachings of Don Juan, Be Here Now.*

In college in Boston we spiraled down into despair, confronting the futility of life as our boyfriends were drafted for a senseless and unjust war. We had no words for our despair, but the word would have been . . . existentialist.

What joy, then, to discover a fresh and more positive formulation of these existential questions from a fellow homeopath:

Am I alone in life or do I act in synchrony with nature and with
  others?
Is my presence in the world sustainable?
Am I oriented in space and time?
Can the boundary between life and death be abided?
Will the insurrection of my birth prove fruitful?

Sages and scholars, poets and philosophers have pondered these questions for millennia. But never before has a system of medicine offered both insight and healing. Homeopathy is like a great chord in music. The physical conditions it addresses form a strong stable foundation, like the bass notes. Psychological conditions and mental deficits comprise the middle octaves of this great mind-body medicine. And in recent years, more esoteric aspects—remedies for karmic bonds and quantum entanglements—have formed a kind of descant as homeopaths pursue the subtle energies. Now Jerry Kantor's *The Emotional Roots of Chronic Illness* reveals a realm of healing that heretofore had been beyond the range of our hearing, as it were: the top notes representing the highest preoccupations of the human spirit.

For the past two hundred years homeopathy has created a strong and solid foundation of proof for its effectiveness, not only for common acute and chronic illnesses but even for the great scourges of humanity—cholera and yellow fever, the plague and Spanish flu. In the homeopathic hospitals and clinics of the nineteenth century, meticulous patient records noted in quaint and crabbed cursive the apparently miraculous cures of homeopathic medicines. (It is only in the twenty-first century that the newly emerging field of ultra-high-dilution physics has begun to reveal the scientific laws behind homeopathy's successes. Like acupuncture, homeopathy worked long before Western science could explain it.)

Meanwhile the nature-cure mental hospitals described in Kantor's *Sane Asylums* successfully used homeopathic medicines more than a century ago to cure mental illnesses that modern psychiatric medications can only hope to palliate. His *Toxic Relationship Cure* details homeopathic medicines to heal emotional wounds from toxic mothers, unfaithful lovers, bullying bosses, and even a very judgmental God.

Homeopathy's founder nearly two centuries ago was a German physician who—disillusioned with the leeches and toxic medicines of his day—studied natural healing systems around the world, including herbs of Europe and the Americas. Samuel Hahnemann's understanding of health in terms of the body's energy system was most likely infused by his questioning of travelers from China and India. And the roots of his thinking went deep, back through Paracelsus to the ancient Greeks.

Now, for the twenty-first century, this visionary book spans psychology, existential philosophy, and Zen Buddhism. Like Samuel Hahnemann, Kantor has grounded his vision in practical applications. To bring his abstract concepts to life, Kantor draws on cases from his practice as well as examples from poetry, art, and mythology. Homeopaths and all those passionate about homeopathy will appreciate how he parallels the five classic miasms (hereditary patterns) of homeopathy with the Five Elements of Chinese Medicine, while providing new uses and new insights into dozens of remedies.

Arsenicum album, for example—one of the most widely used homeopathic medicines, friend of allergy sufferers with drippy noses and travelers with Montezuma's Revenge—holds the existential question, Is my presence in the world sustainable? Arsenicum album has a particular angle on this question: Is my circle of love secure? Fearing death, the Arsenicum album patient hoards resources to ensure her family's survival. Thus, Kantor provides new insight into the well-known anxiety and frugality of the patient needing Arsenicum album.

The wealth of this book is not limited to homeopaths, however; it will benefit psychologists, philosophers, and everyone who has ever pondered "the great questions of Life, Death, God, and the Universe."

BEGABATI LENNIHAN, RN, CCH

BEGABATI LENNIHAN, RN, CCH, is a Harvard graduate and author of *Your Natural Medicine Cabinet* and two other books on holistic health care written under her middle name, Burke. A practicing homeopath for more than twenty years in Cambridge, Massachusetts, she is the former director of two professional training programs in homeopathy and has presented at national and international conventions, including the Integrative Healthcare Symposium.

Acknowledgments

The sensibility that produced *The Emotional Roots of Chronic Illness: Homeopathy for Existential Stress* was shaped by numerous influences. These include readings in philosophy (especially phenomenology), existential psychology, spirituality, Chasidism, Zen Buddhism, Greek mythology, Traditional Chinese Medicine, biomedicine, and of course homeopathy. Though I am blessed to have been instructed by many wonderful teachers, the greatest wellspring of knowledge has always been my patients, for whom healing has regularly entailed their willingness to grapple with life's quandaries. Thanks, too, to my wonderful editors, Jamaica Burns and Abigail Lewis, and to my wife, Hannah, for her support in the writing of this book.

Preface

A dense fog descended as I was driving to work the other day. *With zero visibility, what do I do?* I asked myself. Suddenly less pragmatic, anxiety-laden versions of the question presented themselves: *Where am I? Where am I headed? Do other drivers know I am here? Why has this murk suddenly engulfed me?*

The daily struggle often entails other types of fog: My fiancé of five years has called it quits. *What do I do now?* But then suddenly anguished questions arise: *Have I no worth? Was I a fool all along? Who am I when alone? Will anyone else ever love me? What should I do with my grief and rage?*

The fog can be more challenging when it entails physical survival: If trapped in a war-torn enclave or concentration camp, I ask myself, *How can I obtain food? By what means can my family and I remain alive?*

During an interval of safety the mind poses entirely different questions: *How have I earned this circumstance? On one random day I can be suffering and on another day be well fed and living in luxury—is existence not absurd?*

Even when posed to the masters of divination, answers sought by these questions are difficult to access. The I Ching, Tarot, Egyptian or Celtic runes, and Oracle at Delphi all fling the question back at me, offering at best the description of a spiritual quandary that is mine and mine alone to resolve. The quest for meaningfulness is ingrained, so we might as well admit that at one time or another each of us becomes an existentialist.

Zen master Yunmen once asked: "I'll give you medicine according to your disease. Well, the whole world is medicine plants. Which one is yourself?"[1] He was positing that a core self is accountable for illness and health. Here and in many other teachings the greatest existential query, *Who am I,* is probed. Yunmen's question also challenges doctors: If the aim is to induce healing, first strive to comprehend the human condition. Chiefly homeopaths and a mere handful of physicians take this dictum seriously.

A theme woven through my previous book, *Sane Asylums: The Success of Homeopathy before Psychiatry Lost Its Mind,* is that the advent of psychopharmacological treatment carried with it a theft, that of our birthright to face and learn from the exigencies of existence. In a devilish bargain we acceded to diagnoses of anxiety, depression, psychosis, and any of five types of bipolarity. We accepted in exchange an empty promise that medication would cure all our troubles. The deal cheated us out of opportunities to grapple with existential stress. We could say that psychopharmacology has delimited our potential to evolve.

My notion of existential stress extends beyond what is normally associated with situational disquietude. It encompasses quandaries embedded within our being and becoming. Physical symptoms of existential stress can be rooted in the lineage of a family's struggle with a particular existential issue. Symptoms thereafter epigenetically evoked express illness susceptibility pertaining to the issue, coded within our genetic profile.

As the torment of quandaries induces illness, my intent is to reiterate for homeopaths the existential relevance of their medicines. Other aims include intriguing the educated reader and also, however quixotic, enticing existential psychologists to investigate homeopathy.

In 2021 I volunteered to provide an all-day seminar for the Ontario College of Homeopathic Medicine titled "Existential Quandaries and Their Relation to Chronic Illness." Preparation for the lecture plunged me down a rabbit hole, as this turned out to be a book-length topic.

For many, the case for homeopathy lies in its proffering a reliable, inexpensive, side-effect-free, and nonpharmaceutical recourse to acute illness. While not trivial, this is the least of it. Homeopathy reverses the disease process. Demanding psychologically sophisticated remedy analysis, its power to cure is matter-of-factly assumed by experienced patients and practitioners alike.

Even this is not the whole picture. Homeopathy's relevance extends beyond personality profiling. Many of its medicines embed and therefore address existential themes. This matters because though an existential quandary lacks a logical answer, it contains a tormenting charge, which, if not dispelled, can induce illness.

Though the position does not officially exist, I consider myself a philosopher of medicine, someone whose job description involves unifying medical theory. An early effort produced an integrative medicine text titled *Interpreting Chronic Illness: The Convergence of Traditional Chinese Medicine, Homeopathy, and Biomedicine.* A diagnostic synthesis of Traditional Chinese Medicine (TCM), biomedicine, and homeopathy, the book introduced a method through which the somatic language of chronic illness symptoms could be deciphered. The English language is ill-suited to mind/body state descriptions and so a diagnostic framework was poached from Traditional Chinese Medicine's Five Phases (or Wuxing) system. I repurposed "cyclical" dynamics within the Five Phases model in order for homeopathic remedies and their themes to be schematically depicted.

The resulting synthesis enlarges the scope of Traditional Chinese Medicine and gains homeopathic medicine a feature it lacks. Via introduction of the "generating cycle" dynamic, healthful function can be schematized within homeopathic theory. In 2017 I extended my diagnostic model by correlating TCM's Five Phases with homeopathy's five classical miasms (*Cyclical Remedy Complexes: Their Origin within Traditional Chinese Medicine and Relevance for Miasmatic Theory*). While I was so doing, the five core existential questions presented in this book came to light. Those of us prone to asking *What is the meaning of life?* may find that defusing the charge contained within these five core existential questions provides an answer.

Since that time, remedies embedding subcategories of the five core questions have been identified and organized in accordance with my reformulated Five Phases model and a tool that I call "sense dimensional analysis," in part inspired by David Abram's sense realm exploration, *The Spell of the Sensuous.* Model building invites continual tweaking and so my classifications are neither infallible nor immutable. Remedies chosen comprise a representative but not exhaustive list. The work is ongoing.

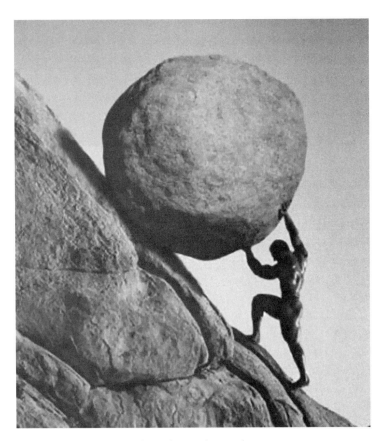

The absurdity of our day-to-day strivings

Introduction

The twenty-first century is a challenging time to be alive. Never before has so much information bombarded us from so many quarters, nor has the future offered so many potentially perilous options. In the face of this a certain amount of angst might be considered a normal response, but when it interferes with daily life it can become intolerable. This book is an effort to address our emotional unrest, the existential stress that can hobble the thoughtful and intelligent response required for an optimally balanced life.

The Emotional Roots of Chronic Illness's topic is the havoc wreaked on body and soul by bedeviling conundrums. A personal, benign bugaboo is the following: It appears I have free will. When the same uniquely "me" life challenge again and again recurs, I find myself asking: *How much of the trajectory of my life is foreordained? To what extent am I entitled to spiritual guidance so that choices I make align with my destiny?* Extra credit will be awarded to the reader helping me out with this.

The reader will encounter a showcasing of the psychological depth of homeopathic remedies. Homeopathy is applicable to existential psychology, health care policy, and human development. It is also a globally popular form of medicine, integral to the health care systems of many countries. According to the World Health Organization homeopathy is the second most widely practiced form of medicine in the world.

Additionally, an integrative medicine vision is offered with therapeutic possibilities that may intrigue the educated reader and the existential psychologist. Existentialist philosophy mines the human condition and its associated quandaries. Its five themes, each of which embeds a health-subverting stress, are:

1. Existence precedes essence. This concerns a disquieting variability within individual consciousness holding sway over greater certainty associated with a conclusive defining of man or woman. Our acts define us, but after we are dead all that remains is an impression left on those who survive us (Jean-Paul Sartre).

2. Within existence a generalized state of anxiety is unavoidable. Faith can be invoked to offset but not displace doubt (Soren Kierkegaard).

3. Existence is inherently absurd, as the myth of Sisyphus suggests. We are condemned to a life of repetitive and ultimately pointless activity comparable to pushing a boulder up a hill only to see it roll down again (Albert Camus). It is absurd also in the tragicomedy of endlessly waiting for some what-have-you that will likely never arrive (*Waiting for Godot* by Samuel Beckett).

4. Existence and also death are predicated on the great void of nothingness. At the same time "unconcealment" of meaning from the void is a nondualistic phenomenon, indicating the meaninglessness of distinguishing between subject and object (Martin Heidegger). Because onus rests upon phenomena rather than subject or object, this position supports the homeopathic approach to case-taking.

5. Human beings are inherently alienated. This can be from God, from societal dictates, or from rationality itself. Individual freedom can thus arise solely from the assumption of personal responsibility or encounter with a mystical force. Will to power can establish freedom (Friedrich Nietzsche); recourse can be taken in will to meaning (Viktor Frankl); or in the face of nothingness, an action in and of itself can do the trick (Jean-Paul Sartre). The philosopher Arthur Schopenhauer held a unique notion of the will according to which alienation not from God but from rational ideas necessarily follows. Schopenhauer's will is a quasi-mystical life force whose nature might be encountered only through aesthetic experience, given that the intellect is of such little use in understanding the world. Schopenhauer's pessimism that reality is inherently unknowable found favor following the ill-fated revolutions of 1848 against European monarchies. These culminated in repression and disillusionment among liberals. Schopenhauer's perspective reverberates

today in existentialism's more dire perspectives as well as in the celebration of art for art's sake.

A correlate of this philosophy is existential psychology, one of whose founders, the Swiss psychiatrist Ludwig Binswanger, reframed what had been considered psychic abnormalities. These he viewed as distortions in a patient's self-image reflecting disorientation within the "lifeworld," a realm of thoughts, feelings, and actions other than the empirical, observation-based world of science.

A latter-day existential psychiatrist is Viktor Frankl. So that lifeworld existence is bearable, Frankl's approach, known as logotherapy, mobilizes an individual's motivation to seek meaning in life. Elaborating on Frankl's notion is the framework of Irvin Yalom, whose impetus to meaning utilizes twelve therapeutic factors: altruism, cohesion, universality, interpersonal learning input and output, guidance, catharsis, identification, family reenactment, self-understanding, instillation of hope, and existential factors.

Holding that the mind and body are inseparable, holistic philosophy correlates mental ailments with physiological symptoms and vice versa. The field of psychology is hamstrung due to having defined itself as limited to nonphysiological mental ideation and emotional stress. Bypassing the subconscious, psychology's tried-and-true methods convey appeals to executive function, a realm within which the charge to attend to reason, modify certain behaviors, recontextualize a situation, exercise willpower, relax or practice acceptance, take up a cause, dredge up past memories, or adopt a spiritual quest is feasible. But apart from forays into hypnosis, neurolinguistic programming, and biofeedback, cooperation from the subconscious mind is not sought.

Homeopathy engages and invokes the subconscious mind. A fully taken case of existential torment featuring constant worry, anxiety, depression, loss of motivation, exhaustion, and diminished social interaction includes physical symptoms that, when interpreted, are windows into subconscious thinking. By signifying an existential ailment's cause, physical symptoms dictate the course of treatment. Astute psychologists and therapists on occasion also take note of physical symptoms. But other than referring the client to a physician, little use of these is made. For most physicians and therapists, acknowledging the subconscious and its pathology is one thing, but the purging of inner demons another matter. Yet homeopathic experience with existentially rooted ailments reveals that the subconscious mind and inherited mindsets are amenable to change.

My overview of homeopathic remedies embodying existential themes is far from comprehensive. There are also remedies that lack an existential issue. For the purposes of this book, existential questions, dilemmas, or quandaries have three characteristics. They are:

- Universal, relating to the human condition
- Deeply ingrained, as in either predating birth or rooted in infancy
- Logically unanswerable

How are existential and nonexistential remedies differentiated?

- Calcarea carbonica, made from oyster shell, is used to treat a huge list of symptoms reflecting metabolic disharmony. What makes Calcarea carbonica existential is the remedy state's reflection of infantile, post-birth vulnerability, as in a naked oyster's yearning for the security and protection of its absent shell. The remedy's core issue of feeling unprotected and overwhelmed by the world is universal and clearly existential.
- When a susceptibility to trauma is ingrained, the lasting effects of acute trauma are not necessarily existential. For example, Arnica montana, used to treat muscular/skeletal trauma, embeds an "I'm okay!" theme. The remedy state reflects a level of consciousness that seeks to escape a compromised body. This is the state of shock, a protective measure serving to insulate us from the full impact of an onerous trauma. Even when long-standing, such trauma is not existential.
- Made from tin, Stannum metallicum reflects a theme described by Jan Scholten pertaining to one's becoming used up or emptied out (a tin can). To the extent that each of us ages and is destined over time to become decreasingly useful, this *is* existential. When a patient enters into the remedy state due to the grief of having actu-

ally been traumatically discarded or treated as an afterthought, this may also *not* be existential.

- Samuel Becket would appreciate a bowel nosode—an ultramolecular homeopathic preparation derived from gut bacterial isolates—made from salmonella. Its related remedy, Dysentery co, is prescribed for the excessive use of antibiotics, endocrine disturbances, and respiratory or gastrointestinal issues. What the existentialist author of *Waiting for Godot* would relate to is the remedy's emotional torment concerning "waiting indefinitely" states.

In the homeopathic perspective, introduced existential stress is reformulated to accommodate its physiological, subconscious, and inherited expression. The third section of Part One of this book presents a remedial but practical model called the Inborn Toolkit of the Emotions.

Following that, a more sophisticated model is introduced. In accordance with Traditional Chinese Medicine and homeopathy's miasmatic theory, robust health is tied to existential viability, whereas failures to defuse five newly identified existential quandaries are shown to induce chronic illness. The quandaries are:

1. Synchrony versus isolation (tubercular miasm). *Am I alone in life or do I act in synchrony with nature and with others?*
2. Challenge versus anxiety (psoric miasm). *Is my presence in the world sustainable?*
3. Centeredness versus disorientation (sycotic miasm). *Am I oriented in space and time?*
4. Consolidation versus entropy (syphilitic miasm). *Can the boundary between life and death be abided?*
5. Creativity versus chaos (cancer miasm). *Will the insurrection of my birth prove fruitful?*

Homeopathic remedies associated with these essential questions and their subcategories are described. Accurately chosen remedies defuse the energetic charge of unresolved core quandaries, thus engineering reversal of chronic illness pathology.

Examples of a core question addressed with a homeopathic remedy include:

- French existentialism deconstructed in terms of subconsciously processed trauma associated with the German occupation of France during World War II. Jean-Paul Sartre's obsession with inauthenticity accounted for via the arborvitae-derived remedy Thuja occidentalis.
- The emotionally impoverished, statistics-obsessed 1950s avatar of nuclear war survival, Herman Kahn, and the iconic mushroom cloud made sense of in terms of sycotic remedies Thuja occidentalis and Natrum sulphuricum.
- Thuja healing a teenage boy in whom a dire existential lesson taught in a high school biology class instigated a delusion that he was a robot.
- Due to their promotion of centeredness overcoming disorientation within the sense dimension of Smell, the value of remedies Verbascum alba and Lapis album in the treatment of frameshift mutation-based cancer of the breast and large intestine.
- The remedies Fluoricum acidum and Petroleum as fitting existential issues bedeviling one-time U.S. president Donald Trump.

The final chapter of this book, "In the Strait of Messina," discusses the existential challenge of thriving into old age. A parallel is made with Ulysses at the end of his long homeward voyage, having to navigate between two hazards, the Scylla of cancer on the one side and the Charybdis of chronic illness on the other. The symbolism of Charybdis, the goddess of the whirlpool, embodies centripetal movement pertaining to chronic illness that the Wuxing's schemata, also known as the Five Phases, serves to illuminate.

In the appendices the reader will find resources for other existential perspectives on homeopathy.

PART ONE

· · · · · · · · · · · · · ·

A Homeopathic Framework

Contextualizing
the Law of Similars

The U.S. Food and Drug Administration (FDA) designates homeopathic medicines as drugs. Although commonly used to resolve acute conditions, homeopathy's most transformative expression is in its constitutional (or classical) form, typically applied for the sake of reversing the course of chronic illness. Constitutional homeopathy is homeopathy at its best, as well as the first and most powerful version of a nanomedical system.

Homeopathy's central dictum, the law of similars (use like to cure like), may be restated: In the appropriate situation, illness or disease symptoms are effectively addressed by a substance whose otherwise toxic effect is to produce equivalent or similar symptoms.

HOMEOPATHY AS ANTIVENOM

A version of the law of similars underlies the production of drugs known as antivenoms. Homeopathic medicines may therefore be compared to antivenom used to counteract snakebite. Here a nonlethal amount of the collected venom of a poisonous snake is injected into a large mammal, such as a horse. By way of combatting the venom's toxicity, the horse's immune system produces antibodies. These are harvested from the horse's blood serum in order to produce the antivenom administered to a human bitten by the same snake. While antivenom for snakebites works only when made from the specific venom, homeopathic medicines have a much broader sphere of action. A homeopathic medicine can be used for any condition similar to one that the full-strength starting substance could create.

BYPASSING THE MIDDLEMAN

. . . Or in this case the middle mammal. Homeopathic medicines can be prepared from a dilution of the same snake venom and directly administered to an individual suffering from symptoms closely akin to those caused by the snakebite. So long as homeopathic medicines are prescribed in accordance with the law of similars, the FDA officially views them as pharmaceuticals, imbuing a status that nutritional supplements and herbs lack.

Commonly known as remedies, homeopathics can address psychological symptoms unrelated to the original starting substance. For example, Natrum muriaticum (or Nat. mur. for short, made from sodium chloride or common table salt) is well known in homeopathy for its ability to release people from silent grief (as in, my husband died and I never shed a tear). How can table salt help with long-held, unexpressed grief?

When table salt—or any substance—is put through the special homeopathic manufacturing process known as "dynamization" or "potentiation," it develops the ability to heal on mental, emotional, energetic, behavioral, and even spiritual levels. It also foments healing of physical conditions untreatable with table salt. In the case of Natrum muriaticum these include conditions of dryness (dry mouth, dry skin) or water retention.

Homeopaths learn which symptoms match each remedy by means of a research methodology called a "proving." A group of healthy people take the remedy in a low potency (more material, less energy) and monitor their responses. Their observations are collected, organized, and ranked in importance so as to become a part of the *materia medica* of the remedy. As homeopaths use it and share their success stories, their clinical experience serves to expand the original materia medica profile. For example, although thyroid conditions did not appear in Natrum muriaticum's proving, over time the medicine was nevertheless found to be effective for thyroid conditions.

SIMILARITY VS. DUPLICATION

The use of the word "like" in the law of similars alludes to something being akin to and not identical. This is because homeopathy requires *similarity* of action, not duplication. When the principle relies on identity rather than similarity, such as in treatment of an actual snakebite with the same snake's toxin, such treatment is designated tautopathy, not homeopathy. An example of tautopathy is when the medicine Rhus radicans works quickly to quell the itching of a skin rash resulting from exposure to the same poison ivy plant that was diluted to make the Rhus radicans remedy.

HOMEOPATHY AS NANO-MEDICINE

Information from the medicinal substance is stored in the water by creating formations like ice crystals or snowflakes, the shape of each one determined by the starting substance. The resulting formations store medicinal information, somewhat like the nanotechnology computer chips that store information in tiny compounds only one molecule wide. The work of Dr. Bell suggests that nano-medicine is epitomized by homeopathy. In her paper "Adaptive Network Nanomedicine: An Integrated Model for Homeopathic Medicine," alternative medicine researcher Iris Bell equates the constituents of homeopathic medicines with miniscule entities known as nanoparticles and nanobubbles.[1] These are shown in low doses to impact biological cells, creating homeostasis or promoting hormetic effects.

REMEDY PRODUCTION

The dilution process renders the medicines safe. (They are diluted to such an extent that according to the laws of conventional chemistry, there should be no molecules of the starting substance in the dilution; cutting-edge research in the realm of ultra-dilution physics has demonstrated that in fact there are molecules even in highly diluted homeopathic remedies.) Continuing developments within science—

for example, the work of the 2008 Nobel Prize–winning virologist Luc Montagnier—indicate that homeopathic effects reflect the ability of water molecules to retain memory of a diluted substance's imprint.[2]

NON-HOMEOPATHIC EXTENSIONS OF THE LAW OF SIMILARS

The law of similars is not the exclusive domain of homeopaths. Vaccines capitalize on the idea of using one pathogen to provoke host immunity to a similar pathogen. Inoculation differs from homeopathy in that vaccines contain a greater amount of the original pathogenic substance. Also, as opposed to homeopathy's customized method, vaccines use a one-size-fits-all approach.

Pediatricians invoke an untoward version of the law of similars when treating hyperactive children with the amphetamine-like drug Ritalin, the brand name for methylphenidate. At least in the short run, Ritalin's stimulant action produces the paradoxical effect of moderating hyperactive behavior. This is due to the drug's being an agonist—a biochemical enabling agent. Ritalin's binding to opiate receptors allows neurotransmitters such as dopamine and norepinephrine to avoid reuptake and linger in the synapse (neuron juncture). Desirable though temporary effects such as euphoria, better hearing, or strengthened focus result. Before long, the drug's antagonistic and less desirable effects, including dazedness, aggression, a sense of being shut off from reality, and addictiveness, start to manifest.

The principle can be found at play outside of medicine. The expression "hair of the dog that bit you" refers to what drinkers do to ameliorate a morning-after hangover—imbibe a dose of the alcoholic beverage that intoxicated them the previous night.

The Law of Similars within Psychology
The law of similars can also be triggered in a nonphysiological context.

Stockholm Syndrome

An act of piracy has lent the name of the ship on which it was perpetrated to a psychological phenomenon known as identification with the oppressor. Its mechanism has broad implications for homeopathic remedy analysis.

Stockholm syndrome is named after a hostage situation in Stockholm in 1973, in which four bank employees bonded with their captors, sided with them against police, and defended them later in court. Psychologists believe that this tendency to identify with someone who is actually abusive, threatening, or dangerous is a coping mechanism in a situation when the victim cannot escape. Stockholm syndrome can also be acquired in consequence of having experienced long-term abuse. Constitutional remedy states thus mirror trauma's effects.

You Can Be Hurt Only at Your Strength

Clinical experience has prompted my adoption of an adage related to Stockholm syndrome's identification with the oppressor phenomenon: "You can be hurt only at your strength." Thus, if someone has been attacked by criticism at a point of weakness, it matters little because the person is uninvested—already weak on that point. The attack fails to alter the target's perspective. For example, you can charge me as being an atrocious needlepoint embroiderer. Go ahead, sue me! I don't care, never having aspired to any such skill! On the other hand, when attacked and overcome at a point of strength, for example in regard to possessing self-confidence, or certitude that specific idealistic values are universal, or skill as a parent, the impact of that attack on my personal strength is more than perspective altering, it is devastating. When one's ingrained mindset—values antithetical to those of a perpetrator—are transformed, the result is not merely agreeable concession; the crushing and supplanting of the victim's values engenders fervent adoption of a kidnapper's or abuser's ideology.

This type of response is also encountered in therapeutic treatment where psychic trauma brought to light reflects the patient's having at some time been crushed at a point of strength. An example is the psyche of someone whose mind, having been subjected to longstanding belittlement by parents or caregivers, buys into their insistence that she is inferior, worthless, stupid, or incompetent. As in Stockholm syndrome, such an individual has adopted as her own the perspective of her oppressors. The situation often calls for the constitutional remedy Thuja to be prescribed.

Prescribe the Symptom

Using like to cure like is exploited within psychology by therapists such as Victor Frankl, Milton Erikson, and their disciples: A "reverse" psychology is employed wherein the same symptom bedeviling a patient is then prescribed (recommended). Utilizing a commonsense principle, the patient is encouraged to exaggerate and wallow in his undesired behavior until its emotional impetus is exhausted and the symptom's *raison d'etre* is no more.

CONSTITUTIONAL DIAGNOSIS

A patient visiting a homeopath with a specific concern, migraine pain for example, may be startled to find the homeopath inspecting him with a wide-angle lens that considers not only his headaches but the totality of his symptoms, behaviors, and even beliefs. This is because additional symptoms—the context surrounding the patient's headaches—provide fertile ground within which the ailment can flourish. Lurking within this fertile ground is a covert issue, an existential question underlying the patient's migraine headache susceptibility. Thus, to return to an earlier example, underlying the Natrum muriaticum remedy state is an existential issue—a question containing powerful emotional charge: *Though the depth of my grief is apparent, I must keep consolation at arm's length. How else to honor the depth of my great loss?* Here we locate the conflict lying at the heart of the patient's migraine headaches.

Finding a Proper Constitutional Remedy

If the effectiveness of a homeopathic medicine hinges on its being accurately prescribed, what then determines its accuracy? The first requirement is that an ideal match between the symptoms we wish to ameliorate and the substance associated with those very same symptoms is found. Invaluable to this matching game is grasping a remedy's essence:

- The practitioner should be able to articulate the remedy's key idea, meaning the specific existential problem with which the patient is grappling and that, via conversion, somaticizes as the patient's symptoms.
- There are characteristic polarities (strengths and weaknesses) within the remedy state (radical disjunct).
- The terrain of action indicates chief mental or emotional features as well as the principal body system or systems affected.

Potentiation

The second requirement is that the substance will have been potentized. A key concept in the preparation of constitutional remedies, "potentized" means that a substance is increased with regard to energy (at the same time that it is lessened with regard to amount). Vigorous shaking (succussion) while systematically diluting the actual substance has been found to heighten the remedy's effect. In its energized, as opposed to materially dense, form, the remedy registers within consciousness at a high level of function. The resulting energized microdosage of our original substance is a homeopathic remedy. A constitutional homeopath specializes in finding a remedy maximally parallel to the patient. To succeed in her quest, the practitioner must scrutinize a terrain encompassing the patient's physical symptoms, cognition (mental features), and affect (characteristic emotional behavior). The homeopath's holy grail is then the similimum, a remedy ideally matching the totality of symptoms exhibited by the patient.

Psychic Excavation

Due to the prominence of *The Myth of Sisyphus,* an essay by the Algerian writer Albert Camus, the title character, who is a god within Greek mythology, has become existentialist ideology's avatar. Beyond being an intellectual icon, Sisyphus has a bodily presence, his tale being that of a man enduring great physical suffering. In the *Iliad* Homer describes an encounter in Hades between Sisyphus and the legendary King Odysseus as follows:

> Aye, and I saw Sisyphus in violent torment, seeking to raise a monstrous stone with both his hands. Verily he would brace himself with hands and feet, and thrust the stone toward the crest of a hill, but as often as he was about to heave it over the top, the weight would turn it back, and then down again to the plain would come rolling the ruthless stone. But he would strain again and thrust it back, and the sweat flowed down from his limbs, and dust rose up from his head.[1]

MINISTERING TO SISYPHUS

According to the Greek myth, Sisyphus, the king of Corinth, was a cunning and ruthless man who managed to cheat death not once, but twice. But then his luck ran out. When Sisyphus perished a third time, an unforgiving Zeus devised a punitive torment whose absurdity, according to Camus, exemplifies man's existential plight.

Sisyphus hates his job. It is repetitious, exhausting, and inane. Updating his resume is not an option. Unimpressed with Sisyphus's

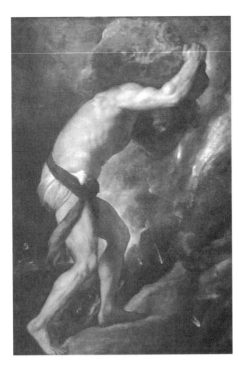

Sisyphus
painted by Titian

efforts and preferring to keep him under his thumb, the boss Zeus won't write a complimentary letter of referral. After laboring for eons, regret for past misdeeds creeps into Sisyphus's mind.

Hope for ameliorating Sisyphus's plight lies with the remedy Germanium metallicum. Individuals needing this medicine abhor their work but feel powerless to make a change and thus continue going through the motions. Germanium metallicum people deny personal implication in their plight since it is always others who are at fault. They themselves, it seems, are misunderstood. Estrangement and out-sider status are their destiny; delusion that life is stagnant becomes self-fulfilling. Misfortune validates a perception that all efforts are in vain. Like Sisyphus, the Germanium metallicum individual is filled with regret. Sisyphus, being a god, is condemned to suffer eternally, while his luckier mortal counterpart, someone who qualifies for Germanium metallicum, will achieve the relief afforded by death. Toward that end, muscular problems and exhaustion will engulf him. Cancer, anemia, diabetes, paralysis, or gastrointestinal issues may be his undoing.

By dispelling a delusion that work is stagnating and rote, a prescription of Germanium would forestall this physical decline. Under the remedy's influence an awareness will dawn of personal culpability for things that have gone wrong. Energy will return. Communication skills will improve or it will appear that others have mysteriously come to understand him better. Before describing how, as opposed to Sisyphus, an actual patient responded to Germanium, a few words about what a remedy achieves are in order.

Psychic Excavation and Pendulum Swing

Homeopathy entails psychic excavation. Once a client "graduates" from an effective remedy it is usually evident that an "onion skin" remedy-state layer has been peeled away. Seemingly an out-of-the-frying-pan-into-the-fire experience, the transition is found meaningful since an underlying layer's core issues and pertaining symptoms are now accessible for treatment. Some of these symptoms will overlap with the previous remedy; others will be new. Symptoms and behaviors arise indicating a drastic polarity shift that I liken to a pendulum swing.

Upon release of its potential energy a pendulum swings past the midpoint of its arc. The pendulum's movement eventuates in a point diametrically opposed to where it started. Similarly, rather than merely reducing the magnitude of an existential issue's charge (a pendulum unaccountably halting at the midpoint of its arc), a dramatic polarity shift in a client's psyche is evident. Liberation from the prior remedy's existential issue is signaled by the pendulum swing. This indicates that regardless of how good a remedy was, a new medicine is called for rather than repeating the old one.

Case Study

Psychic Excavation with a Sisyphus-like Patient

My Sisyphus-like client reported detesting a job to which he felt chained. Though repetitious and pointless, the job "paid the bills." He much regretted educational and career decisions that had led him to his occupational plight. Despite being well-off and possessed of various skills, he felt powerless to quit or even to look around for something else. "Let's say I did?" he asked. "The new job would be no better than the one I have now, likely even worse." In his relationships he felt misunderstood and powerless to do anything about it. I gave him Germanium metallicum.

The conclusion of the remedy's several-weeks-long time frame indicated that psychic excavation was underway. As opposed to griping about his job, he now had a new complaint. Though drained of motivation to look for different work—or to do anything, for that matter—he revealed an upsurge of self-awareness and personal agency in our next session. My client spoke of anguish regarding his dysfunctional family of birth, of its gradual fracturing into multiple indifferent relationships. He reported an unrealistic desire to gain membership in someone else's large family that he recognized as being compensatory.

Surfacing also was a feeling of being unmoored, floating with no sense of being anywhere, that indicated a pendulum swing: As opposed to being chained (in relation to his work), the opposite was now true. He became suddenly *too* free—untethered, disconnected, unmoored. This accounted for his lack of motivation and called for a different remedy, one fitting the new symptoms. My choice was Amethyst immersion derived from a precious gem of the same name and whose themes Peter Tumminello has wonderfully brought to light.[2]

Following Amethyst immersion my client not only gained his footing but in another pendulum swing transitioned from being unmoored into an opposite state. At our follow-up he presented as tethered to material goals. His suddenly raging ambition, intensity, and loquaciousness prompted my prescribing Lachesis muta, a remedy made from the venom of the Brazilian bushmaster snake (whose sycotic "ego versus id" issue is discussed in chapter 3).

In his analysis of the remedy Osmium metallicum Jan Scholten offers an alternative appropriation of the Sisyphus myth. A stage 8 metal situated close to the midpoint of the gold series on the periodic table of the elements, Osmium metallicum, both for good and for ill, represents nearly the zenith of the weighty responsibility theme of the gold series. In this reading Sisyphus, bulling his way to the heights, cannot quite reach them. The tragic theme—"failure through dictatorial behavior"—expresses a downfall resulting from arrogance and ambition, when the pressure to rise becomes implosive and/or attracts opposition.[3]

Condemned to push a huge boulder up a hill, Sisyphus imparts superhuman effort to his task. He succeeds in propelling the boulder upward, almost surmounting the hill's crest before the treacherous rock escapes his grip and careens back down the hill. In its endless repetition Sisyphus's task demands superhuman determination and strength.

As Scholten notes, conditions attached to Osmium metallicum's existential issues include:

Problems with testes and ovaries: inflammation, cancer, cryptorchidism (undescended testes), sterility, amenorrhea, metrorrhagia (irregular uterine bleeding)

Afflictions of bones: necrosis

General inflammation: paralysis, Parkinson's, multiple sclerosis, cancer, headache, swelling of the face

Eye complaints: visual disturbances, glaucoma

Heart ailments: high blood pressure, infarction, congestion of blood, cerebral hemorrhage, anemia

Stomach problems

Whether providing Sisyphus with Germanium metallicum or Osmium metallicum, postal service and Amazon couriers will likely balk: "Make that delivery? No way in hell!"

MINISTERING TO BARTLEBY THE SCRIVENER

Sisyphus's corrective, confining, and severe punishment reflected the respect that Zeus held for the former king's power and the havoc of which Sisyphus remained capable. Sisyphus maintained a formidable presence. When the cards of life are dealt, a hand opposite to that of Sisyphus's can also be held.

Suppose an awareness dawns that *I am obsolete and altogether powerless*. What if the individual's endeavors have become inconsequential, rendering them a nonentity? Whether or not objectively true, such a mindset invokes Bismuth subnitricum, a remedy occupying a tail-end position (stage 15) within the periodic table's gold series, whose theme is power. As an emblem of this state we find the protagonist of a short story by Herman Melville, "Bartleby, the Scrivener: A Story of Wall Street." The scrivener Bartleby is a type of clerk, a copyist, who refuses to perform the sort of writing demanded of him. In response to any request he obstinately repeats, "I prefer not to." The narrator of "Bartleby, the Scrivener" casts back to when Bartleby first came to work for him. It was a time in the 1840s when the wealthy magnate John Jacob Astor owned a great deal of New York City real estate and unrest was rife among the working class. With the Industrial Revolution prompting drastic changes in working conditions, Karl Marx and Friedrich Engels published *The Communist Manifesto* in 1848, calling for revolt among industrial workers. In the United States factory workers did strike, protesting the long hours they worked for low pay. Workers engaged in bookbinding, upholstering, shoemaking, and tailoring engaged in strikes. Rather than stage organized rebellions, white-collar workers on the brink of becoming obsolete could mount passive-aggressive, existential insurrections like the one made by Bartleby.[4]

Bismuth subnitricum's physical symptoms include swollen glands, inflammation, necrosis, weakness, Parkinson's disease, headache, eye pain and diminished vision, gastritis, ulcers, cancer, vomiting, and abdominal pain. Within the extremities a sensation of glowing heat in the thighs can be experienced. Males in need of the remedy are prone to testicular problems and infertility. Females in need of the remedy are likewise prone to infertility, in addition to ovarian issues.[5]

MINISTERING TO HAMLET, PRINCE OF DENMARK

An instructive junior version of the Sisyphean "getting to the top is brutal" theme is exemplified by a different remedy. Positioned not within the gold series but in the first quarter (stage 5) of the ferrum series, whose overall concern is our relation to work or the task at hand, we have Vanadium. The Vanadium individual is a perfectionist perfectly aware that the job needs to be done. Doing it exactly right will elevate him, but fear of both failure and success torments him. Rather than Sisyphus, the exemplar is Shakespeare's Hamlet, prince of Denmark. Hamlet knows monstrous evil would be redressed if his murderous uncle could be dispatched. Instead of taking action, Hamlet muses over an existential question: "To be or not to be?" He procrastinates; accidentally kills an elderly advisor to the king, Polonius; dithers; and torments both his girlfriend and himself with riddles.

Case Study
Vanadium and Fear of Fear Itself

One of my clients, a down-to-earth, hardworking woman, has a child with Down syndrome, also in my care, who at birth had numerous health issues. As is often the case the child's immediate state had an impact on the mother's state of health. In the interval following favorable remedy outcomes for both daughter and mother, the mother appeared in my office in an excited state but also agitating about the future. When she reported feeling cold with congested sinuses and expressing the following, I gave her a dose of Vanadium, from which she apparently benefited as shown by this journal entry:

> *Just of late everything has changed for me. The pain is so much better, but it took a while. The panicky stuff is also about through. I just realized I am not going to die. But remaining is still a little doubt in my mind—what if I die tomorrow? I don't want to waste my time on this work [meaning her job]. This feels so existential. I don't want to die before I do something greater or bigger. Oh my God, what is it I want to do with my life? I am ready to climb to the top of the mountain, but where do I want to go next? My fear is of fear, in the back of my head. It's not paralyzing, more just a thought, like my dad is getting older, maybe I should go to Mexico to see him. I don't want to miss out on my parents, because who*

*knows. I don't want to waste my time. I'm needing to find roots with my family, but scared of flying. I want to make a meaningful trip but **am fearful of it**.*

The Vanadium prescription discharged her existential complaint, returning to her a sense of clear purpose.

When presenting with severe physical symptoms a Vanadium candidate may report eye problems, throat pain, coughing up small lumps of bitter yellow and green mucus, stomach and bowel problems, degeneration of the liver, cancer, constipation, ovarian pain, or sciatica. The remedy is also of value in the treatment of anorexia or bulimia.[6]

MINISTERING TO THE CHARACTER PHIL CONNORS OF THE FILM *GROUNDHOG DAY*

The chief protagonist of the existentialistic comedy *Groundhog Day* is Phil Connors, played by actor Bill Murray. Connors is a jaded television weatherman assigned to report on the annual Groundhog Day event in Punxsutawney, Pennsylvania. With no accounting for how this comes about, Connors is ensnared in a time loop compelling him to relive February 2 over and over again. The film enmeshes Connors in the mindset of the remedy Gallium metallicum by not only refusing to release him from the routine of his everyday work, but by ruthlessly exaggerating its deadly repetitiveness.

Evocative of the played-out state, Gallium metallicum's symptoms include a sense of failure, fear of falling, paralysis, criticism, opposition, and anticipation of being observed. Dreams associated with Gallium metallicum may involve crime, murder, futile efforts, and being paralyzed. Physical complaints associated with the remedy include cancer (particularly of the bladder or cervix), paralysis, a feeling of the eyes being glued together, blockage of the ears and deafness, anemia, stomach issues, nausea, vomiting, diabetes, Paget's disease, and psoriasis.[7]

Case Study
....

Gallium metallicum for the
Rigors of Repetitive Responsibilities

A client of mine who had become exhausted and jaded from the rigors of repetitive nursing responsibilities reported her feelings:

> Am just barely strong enough to do what I do. So very tedious to do four-layer bandage wraps on people, very tedious, just barely able to do it. Experiencing a tremendous amount of anxiety. Overwhelmed by all the preparation the work entails. Ears blocked, no desire to eat. This is so unlike me, I've always been masterful at my work.

Following a course on Gallium she returned, at which time she reported an unblocking of her ears as well as the regaining of her energy. As opposed to complaining of barely holding on, she now wished only not to be interfered with when doing her work.

MINISTERING TO DOUGLAS FAIRBANKS
AND CHARLIE CHAPLIN

So far we have seen the theme of being physically and emotionally played out in action within the gold series with respect to power (Germanium metallicum, Osmium, and Bismuth nitricum) and also in the ferrum series pertaining to work (Vanadium and Gallium metallicum). A remedy from the silver series whose primary theme is creativity is now referenced. Occupying a near tail-end (stage 15) position amidst silver's row on the periodic table is Tellurium metallicum, a remedy representative of and curative to the problem of being creatively outmoded.

According to Jan Scholten: "They feel that their creations are no longer accepted by the general public. They have come to the end of their career and it is only the goodwill of the people that keeps them going. They are not taken seriously anymore. They don't take themselves seriously either, but still get very angry when they are not being accepted or understood. This feeling often comes about after several big projects have failed."[8]

Tellurium's conditions, according to Scholten, encompass cancer; weakness; neuralgia, neuropathy, and demyelization of the nerve fibers; vertigo; and headache, specifically above the left eye.

There are numerous eye symptoms including inflammation of the iris, choroidal or conjunctival damage, infiltrations, cataract, pterygium, lachrymation, and visual disturbance.

Ear symptoms include infections (a strong indication), such as those producing watery and stinking yellow, gray, or green discharges that smell like rotten fish. The discharges can be acrid, sharp, itchy, or radiating painfully toward the throat and could cause loss of hearing.

Additional symptoms Scholten outlines include:

Mouth symptoms such as garlic breath or a metallic taste
Throat symptoms—expelling mucus from the nose; hoarseness (strong feature), loss of voice, stammering
Various ailments of the lungs
Stomach symptoms—pain, heartburn, nausea, feeling empty and weak, faintness
Injuries of the liver
Problems with testes and genitalia among males
Problems with ovaries and genitalia among females
Urine that smells of ammonia
Back pain, with the spine feeling tender to the touch or as if the back has been broken
Sciatica (a prominent symptom)
Skin symptoms—ringworm, eczema on hands and feet, ears, or occiput[9]

In my own practice a typical Tellurium case might involve a serious equestrian falling from a horse and developing sciatica that made it impossible to compete in equestrian events.

Tellurium metallicum could well have been prescribed for ailments due to stresses endured by silent-screen movie stars who for the first time had to encounter the challenge of working in the talkies. Here are two examples:

The swashbuckling Douglas Fairbanks was a major star of the silent film era. The advent of early sound films put a damper on his enthusiasm for filmmaking. At the same time that motion pictures were changing, the actor's athletic abilities and general health also underwent decline, exacerbated by his being a chain-smoker. As Petruchio in a 1929 "talkie" of Shakespeare's *The Taming of the Shrew* and in subsequent sound films he was poorly received by Depression-era audiences. Though he continued to hang on in the film industry, Fairbanks died young, of a heart attack at age fifty-six.

For Charlie Chaplin the Great Depression likewise posed a challenge. His 1931 silent film *City Lights* earned him critical acclaim and audiences. But *City Lights* was also a unicorn, a lone silent film in the brave new world of sound films. At the time Chaplin could not fathom incorporating speech into his films. His comedy was steeped in physical humor and he could not conceive how speech would improve it. Fearing he was about to become yesterday's news, Chaplin grew lonely and despondent and considered relocating to China. Unsure of where his career was headed, Chaplin left the country for sixteen months to clear his head. He returned with a new paramour, actress Paulette Goddard, and weathered his Tellurium-themed crisis by exploiting other talents—musical composition and writing. With the making of his masterwork *Modern Times,* Chaplin transitioned brilliantly and on his own terms into the new era.

Our Inborn Toolkit
of Five Emotions

In Traditional Chinese Medicine's Five Phase theory, a rudimentary psychological model is presented within which five basic emotions, each of which is aligned with a particular phase, are contained: Joy aligns with Fire, anxiety (or worry) aligns with Earth, sadness (or grief) aligns with Metal, fear aligns with Water, and anger aligns with Wood.

The pared-down model undergoes elaboration throughout this book. For the moment it is the basis for a practical metaphor in my Inborn Toolkit of the Emotions. The point is made that when likening each basic emotion to a tool, an emotion's expression serves the purpose of problem solving. After an issue has been resolved, as with a physical tool, the emotion can be put away, on reserve for a future problem. Dallying with or overemploying an emotion, similar to hanging on to an unused tool, serves no purpose (unless one is an actor). Similarly, refusal or reluctance to employ a needed tool or emotion impedes and complicates interpersonal transaction.

Therapeutic recourse to emotional tools is easy to recommend; seeing that the directive is carried out is another matter. This is because emotions we employ while coping are not consciously accessed. Our reactions—individualized "default" response patterns—release automatically from the subconscious. Even when clearly self-sabotaging, dysfunctional response patterns are difficult to rework and routinely defeat the finest therapists. On the other hand, because it operates behind the scenes, as it were, the directive of a well-chosen remedy is not easily ignored. The remedy is like a bomb deposited within the subconscious, one that, after its explosion, the dust having settled and the air cleared, leaves a transformed inner terrain. With the psychic landscape altered, interest in the Inborn Toolkit's possibilities is refreshed.

Imagine a tradesman with five tools in his kit. These are a sketchpad, a screwdriver, pliers, a hacksaw, and a hammer. Suppose he were to venture forth on a gig thinking, "Today I'm going to use only my screwdriver." Or suppose he declares, "I hate my hammer. Today I'm just not going to use it." This would be unlikely. A tradesman worth his salt respects all his tools, each of which he uses according to his needs, and each of which he places back in his toolkit when an allotted task is completed.

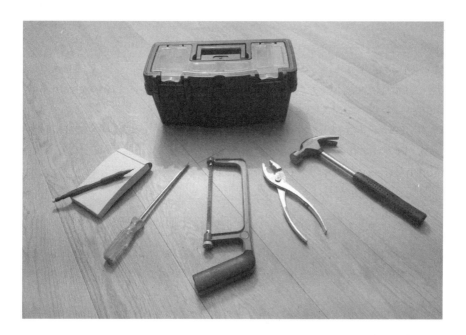

Proper utilization of an emotional tool is cathartic, meaning a satisfactory outcome is poised to result. Just as we are engineered with a pathogen-resisting immune system, so are we also from birth equipped with an emotional set of tools, each of which enables repair of a broken situation or renovation of a shabby state of affairs. Over- or underuse of any one emotional tool is bad workmanship, causing the framework of the psyche to wobble.

Before describing these tools, we note that our emotional tools can do a lot, but only within reason. A standard toolkit might be used to build a shed in the backyard, but we don't expect to build a skyscraper with it. Similarly, trauma or abuse occurring in childhood when our emotional tools are not yet fully honed is challenging to overcome. Traumatic events debilitate our tools, damaging our ability to cope. Or, as in the phenomenon of denial, a tool can fall into disuse.

Though generally desirable, a state of tranquility does not indicate the absence of toolkit emotions. Rather, what tranquility can signal is secure awareness of our toolkit's availability, of its readiness at hand.

It is said that a sixth foundation emotion is disgust. When discussing sense dimensional modeling, the expression of disgust, because it possesses little relevance to existential stress, will be viewed as an amalgam of core emotions.

The sequence in which the tools are presented reflects a progressive development within TCM's cyclically arranged Five Phases. The cycle's clockwise directionality models a healthful dynamic known as the Generating cycle, which will receive close attention in our discussion of the five sense dimensions.

THE SKETCHPAD OF JOY

It is such a joy to view the big picture when the blueprint of a project is envisioned and everything is hanging together. We see it in its entirety. Now the time arrives when what exists on paper must be actualized. The glory of its vision must give way to the drudgery of execution. Dwelling forever in joy is not possible. An individual lost in visions or prone to excess of ego has not learned to put away his sketchpad.

A homeopathic remedy known to upend this applecart is Sulphur. The Sulphur individual is full of inadequately consolidated ideas. The individual is a kind of mad scientist, with a strong ego that hungers for approval. The Sulphur state can be compared to having an inefficient interior metabolic furnace. This metaphor has currency within TCM in the theoretical construct known as the Middle Burner, the furnace-like organs (Spleen and Stomach) that are the heart of the digestive system. The Sulphur individual is always hungry, gassy, aggravated by heat, and prone to skin conditions erupting from the inner "furnace" source. A major remedy (or polycrest—a remedy that affects all or nearly all tissues of the body), Sulphur is one of homeopathy's greatest contributions to medicine.

The Sulphur state can either reflect or promote a dietary issue related to exorphins. Derived from foods, exorphins are opioid peptides available in casein and gluten. Once in the body they activate endorphins and trigger a reward system in the brain involving dopamine release. Because exorphins cause pleasure and prompt euphoria, bread, pasta, and cereal rich in exorphins addict children to these very foods. In order to control excess stimulation the brain produces dopamine. When overly habituated to this demand, capacity to produce dopamine diminishes. Reduced dopamine levels in the body then prompt production of cortisol, the hormone that is primarily responsible for increasing bloodstream sugar in response to stress. Disruption of the reward system engenders endorphin resistance that, in a vicious cycle, then ramps up craving for more gluten.

As I am portraying Sulphur as an existential remedy, let me revisit what is meant by "existential."

Existential quandaries (also known as dilemmas or conundrums) are not just about survival. They have three features:

1. Their issues are universal, meaning they relate to the human condition.
2. They are ingrained, as in either predating birth or being rooted in infancy.
3. They pose a question that is logically unanswerable.

Sulphur satisfies the criteria. It is both universal and rooted in infancy; each one of us was once an infant and the remedy is found to come up often for children. Why this is so has less to do with pathology than with the healthful side of the remedy picture. Sulphur features age-appropriate solipsism (a self-importance, as in *I am the center of the world*); extreme curiosity about surroundings; insistence on being appreciated for the many notions on the child's emotional sketchpad; and an outsized

appetite. Still, when for example gastric problems, asthma, or skin eruptions crop up or if the individual is messy, a grumbler, someone who tends
to slump in chairs when sitting, and displays aversion to bathing, the remedy is invoked. Symptoms arise in consequence of stress associated with
luxuriating in one's sketchpad, not putting it away, so that carrying out
its wonderful ideas can be implemented. Instead, the Sulphur individual
is stuck on a logically unanswerable question: *How am I to be appreciated
for my wonderful ideas when bountiful expression of my acuity is off-putting
to others?*

Soon we shall see how this question represents a subset of a bigger
question discussed within our more elaborate, sense dimensional model:
Is my presence in the world sustainable? There, instead of with the Fire
phase, Sulphur is found positioned within the Earth phase, associated
with what in homeopathy is called the psoric miasm. Homeopathy's
founder, Samuel Hahnemann, held that the psoric miasm (referring
to what he called the primordial itch) gave birth to the other miasms
sycosis and syphilis. For that reason sulphur, the periodic table element
most closely associated with psora, is known as the king of all polycrests
(major remedies).

Let us consider someone whose sketchpad is crumpled and jumbled
within the toolbox. Disappointment and resentment have smudged the
big picture, the overriding blessings of her life. Overwrought, depressed,
and unclear as to where she is in life, she will find a remedy such as Sepia
appropriate. Within Sepia a state of stagnation has taken hold, relegat-
ing her to a limbo betwixt optimism and despair. Though invested in
hope, she has experienced hope to be toxic, and thus her psyche orches-
trates a stagnation of metabolism and blood motility.

THE SCREWDRIVER OF ANXIETY

Imagine you are starving while lost in a wilderness and spy a mushroom.
Eating it will either poison or nourish you. The screwdriver of anxiety
tightens, heightening situational focus. Your hands sweat and your mouth
goes dry as you lift the mushroom toward your mouth. But suddenly
anxiety constrains the impulse. Elevated performance due to anxiety—

here, eschewing a poisonous foodstuff or the partaking of a miniscule nibble—has saved your life. Reluctance to use the screwdriver of anxiety stokes recklessness. A reckless individual can require a homeopathic remedy such as Medorrhinum. Medorrhinum is the nosode derived from gonorrhea and so the individual needing it infuses personal interests with passion and a tendency to go to extremes. Such behavior is related to the gonorrheal miasm known as sycosis and will be discussed in greater detail later. For now, let it suffice that the Medorrhinum individual has diminished use for the screwdriver of anxiety. Among features of the state, the individual is prone to be a night person, is drawn to the ocean, may have familial heart disease, and can lose her train of thought midsentence.

Excessive use of the screwdriver of anxiety, on the other hand, is incapacitating. A homeopathic remedy to diminish excessive anxiety is Arsenicum album. Arsenicum album people are fastidious, perfectionistic, death obsessed, worried about anyone within their circle of love, concerned about aging, and prone to exhaustion.

THE HACKSAW OF SADNESS (OR GRIEF)

The bond was strong between you and your beloved grandmother; now she is gone. Or, once solid, your five-year relationship with your partner is broken. Have you wept to a point of catharsis? Grieved the loss to completion so that you can move on? If not, the hacksaw of sadness (or grief) has yet to cut: Despite an appropriate interval's passage, the bond is not severed and grief remains locked in place. You are sad but unable to cry. This calls for the homeopathic remedy Natrum muriaticum, made from sodium chloride. Natrum muriaticum individuals are self-contained. Compare them to a country that sends all its resources to the periphery. The impression given of studied calm and self-reliance disguises a tenderness of feeling and vulnerability sequestered in the interior. Such a person will cry only in private, be averse to consolation, crave intimacy but keep it at arm's length. Recourse to the hacksaw expresses the unthinkable: *If I cry it would be forever. To complete my grief for this loss would be to dishonor its magnitude.*

Overuse of the hacksaw of sadness, on the other hand, suggests the remedy Pulsatilla nigricans for someone who cries at the drop of a hat. No matter how fervently the loss is sawed away at, the blade fails to cut through and sever it. Never unpacked baggage, longstanding or subconscious memory of having been previously abandoned, makes the effort futile. The Pulsatilla nigricans individual is often a stereotypically "hormonal" woman, or if a boy, seldom older than the age of twelve. The individual has a soft temperament. Your heart goes out to this person.

THE PLIERS OF FEAR

Idioms reliably express the truth. As an example, it is said that fear grips us. As if clasped by pliers, we freeze before taking action. The pliers of fear allow a grasp of the situation and enable an expeditious choice between fighting and fleeing. When the pliers of fear do not lessen their grip, a routine nonthreatening situation can escalate to life-or-death proportions. This may call for the homeopathic remedy Veratrum album. A Veratrum album individual overuses the pliers of fear due to having in the past experienced a sudden loss of social position. Some shocking event has pulled the rug out from under this person and left a feeling of having been abruptly evicted from Paradise. By way of compensation the individual becomes self-righteous. "So lost, only they know the way," describes this peculiar conundrum, a state featuring weakness, sudden vomiting, cold sweat, collapse, and distorted perception. The abrupt onset of weakness in the remedy picture serves to reenact the precipitating "rug pulled out from under me" trauma.

On the other hand, someone in whom fear has inculcated an escapism reaction may become audacious and insensitive to pain. Incapable of finding coping pliers, this individual needs homeopathic Opium. The lack of reactivity within an Opium state features constipation, deep sleep with intense dreaming and snoring, and a feeling of inner tremor.

THE HAMMER OF ANGER

A situation arises requiring immediate and forceful action. Insulted or frustrated, the individual pulls out the hammer of anger and smashes down. Better, but in the same spirit, this force is directed into a creative action. The individual failing to do so fears that natural expression of anger will go badly and culminate in loss of control or violence, so indignation is suppressed. When the individual needing the remedy Staphisagria flies into rageful passion, it is frustrated displacement rather than a cathartic anger that is vented. Such an individual will likely throw an object, slam a door, or weep in frustration, wielding the hammer but using the incorrect end of the tool to claw out a crooked nail. This is anger's dysfunctional cousin vexation, a state featuring repression and trembling with frustration. Overinvested in honor, in the wake of genuine anger the Staphisagria individual would feel worse, not better, which is why the emotion of anger is suppressed in the first place.

Due to social conditioning women are often brought up to "be nice." Women, therefore, tend to require Staphisagria more often than men. However, a male may occasionally need this remedy; the following case study provides an example from my own experience.

Case Study
Staphisagria and the Hammer of Anger

While transitioning a number of my clients from acupuncture to homeopathic care, I wrote an article containing an early version of some of the ideas presented in this book. Despite my having been a homeopath for only a year, a prestigious medical journal accepted my modeling of homeopathic materia medica utilizing TCM-derived schema. I was pleased to hear that no editorial changes were needed and that it would be published in the forthcoming issue. When the issue was released, however, it did not include my article. The editors apologized, assuring me no worries, the issue had in fact been filled but my article would appear in the following issue. Once again, an issue absent my article was published and I received an apology. When the same thing happened once or twice more, pains commenced to visit and radiate down my left arm. My wife, concerned that I might be having a heart attack, sent me to the emergency room, where an EKG found no evidence of heart trouble. Compelled to maintain a dignified front before wonderful journal editors who, after all, were only doing the best they could, but sorely vexed, I had been tearing at myself with the claw end of the hammer. My frustration had evoked the symptom. Despite being miserable at self-prescribing, I ventured a dose of Staphisagria 200C. When the next journal issue was released, my article was included. Its appearance magically coincided with the conclusion of the remedy's time frame and the disappearance of my symptoms.

The Staphisagria state's investment in honor and not utilizing the hammer of anger reflects or promotes injury to an individual's integrity. Harmed inner integrity promotes weakness of the teeth and subsequent tooth decay. Here is how it works: The teeth are the one place in the body where our bones are visible. Everything "hangs" on the skeletal structuring of our bones. They are the physical embodiment of our integrity. Injury to our inner integrity undermines the teeth, whose gleaming white appearance is a billboard advertising our "external" integrity in the guise of aesthetic and sexual appeal (or viability). That a congenital dental issue can reflect a legacy of injured inner integrity is suggested by my experience with a child whose adult teeth failed to erupt and whose baby teeth therefore lingered in place. My aim not to treat the teeth specifically was carried out as my young patient responded well to Staphisagria.

Someone can become enamored of, and overuse, the hammer of anger. The individual with a hair-trigger temper who is instantly provoked into rage will need a remedy such as Stramonium. Here we find a classical post-traumatic stress disorder (PTSD) prescription for the veteran freshly returned from military combat. Such persons are plagued by nightmares of violence, prone to religious beseeching, fear the dark, and are excited by the stimuli of glittering objects. Likewise children who have witnessed terrifying violence and become prone to rage and violent tantrums—a survival response countering fear of abandonment or impending annihilation—will benefit from this remedy.

PART TWO

Five Existential Questions

And Their Corresponding Miasms,
Sense Dimensions, Phases,
Emotions, and Organs

1

Am I alone in life or do I act in synchrony with nature and with others?

*Tubercular Miasm • Touch • Fire Phase •
Joy • Heart–Small Intestine*

When an army of ants crosses a stream the lead ants think nothing of drowning themselves so that their stacked corpses can serve as a bridge for pursuant ants. The behavior of martyr ants is synchronous with the needs of the colony. Human beings, too, must resolve synchrony versus isolation dilemmas: Soldiers march into battle knowing they may be cannon fodder; Russian workers knew they would absorb lethal levels of radiation when acting to secure the melting-down Chernobyl atomic energy plant; at times parents and teachers die for the sake of children in their care. The everyday experience of being ill, too, can raise the question: *Do I quarantine myself with a contagious illness? Shall I accept a vaccine I oppose for the sake of others? I own a petrochemical plant whose revenue puts food on my family's table; shall I renounce this lucrative business to reduce my carbon footprint?* Collapse of the barrier between myself and others can also be joyous, as in the spontaneous elation of slipping into synchrony with nature.

Am I in synchrony? This question lies at the core of what I have

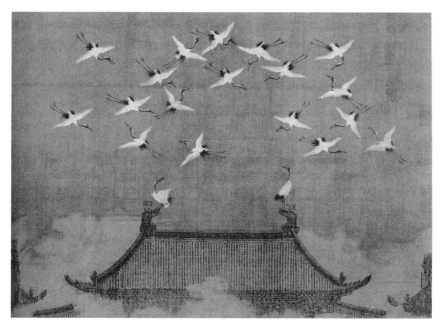

Auspicious Cranes handscroll, Emperor Huizong, Liaoning, Provincial Museum, Shenyang

termed the sense dimension of Touch. It underlies an inborn suscepti-bility to the tubercular miasm as well.*

THE TUBERCULAR MIASM AND THE SENSE DIMENSION OF TOUCH

According to Hahnemann there were three original miasms: psora, syco-sis, and syphilis. Once it became clear that tuberculosis was also a miasm, debate sprang up as to how to account for it. Some of Hahnemann's disciples held that it was psora combined with syphilis. Others decided that it stemmed from sycosis and syphilis. I will explore the question in greater detail shortly. In brief, the feeling of the tubercular miasm can

---

*Providing context for an understanding of specific chronic illness conditions, an expanded discussion of the sense dimension of Touch and of the other four sense dimensions and core dilemmas is offered in the author's *Interpreting Chronic Illness: The Convergence of Traditional Chinese Medicine, Homeopathy, and Biomedicine.*

be described as originating from the suffocating effect of an encroaching and potentially lethal infection. The individual longs to escape from the scourge's proximity. A desperate struggle for freedom ensues whose creative outlet is a response to a sense that the life force is burning its way through the individual. The hyperactive state promotes or reflects suspicion of those close to the individual as well as conditions including respiratory complaints, heart ailments, and deforming arthritis.

The Sense Dimension of Touch

> **Wuxing phase:** Fire
> **Emotion:** Joy
> **Organ:** Heart–Small Intestine (blood circulation)
> **Theme:** Synchrony vs. isolation

Of all the sense organs, touch—the realm of sensations conveying pressure, heat, cold, torque, and pain—has the widest expanse. Not merely a passive receptor reporting conditions on the skin, touch is the will to know and to be known, to commune and to communicate. By conveying the feel of others, touch bridges separation. Martin Buber spoke of an "I-thou" relationship in which the kinship of the self and other is acknowledged. Being in touch constitutes a call with sensory inputs as the response. Individual contractions and relaxations of the heart and the cyclical departures and returns of circulating blood are physiological call and response. When call and response is most meaningful, the heart has been touched. We deem moving poems, films, stories, and conversations touching. A DePauw University study published in August 2009 indicates that touch between persons previously unknown to one another could accurately convey a specific emotion from one to the other.[1]

The rhythm of periodic call and response constitutes a cycle and the phenomenon of circulation. The theme of a great return is suggested when seasonal rains seep into a river and return to the sea or when, drawn by a homing instinct back to ancestral places, herds and flocks undertake epic migrations.

Not all circular patterns are beneficial. Interruption of a healthful cycle, the negation of essential return, can spur acute or chronic illness. Breakdown in touch informs us of otherness and the not-self. Heralding failure of call and response, a divide of separateness forms that can widen into a chasm of isolation wherein anxiety and heartbreak are fostered. Due to its characteristic self-deception and circularity, a pattern of thinking we will later associate with the syphilitic miasm is as treacherous as the whirlpools of Charybdis.

Surprisingly Not Touch Related

Despite mediating sensations of touch, skin diseases are not, according to TCM, particularly Touch related. It is the Lungs rather than Touch's circulatory system cohort that we associate with skin diseases. This is because TCM's physiological functions often reflect ontogeny: In a zygote (embryonic cell) responsibility for the exchange of gases, meaning respiration, is carried out by the cell's membrane (outer skin). Since in a fully developed human being detoxification continues to be carried out by the skin, Lung function pertains to dermatology. Confirming this relationship, acupuncture points on the Lung meridian and the Large Intestine meridian (the large intestine organ itself being composed of skin tissue) are chiefly utilized in the treatment of skin ailments.

Neurological disorders affecting the various touch receptors also do not pertain to the sense dimension of Touch. Within TCM they are more closely related to the Kidneys when their locus is the central nervous system or to the Liver when their locus is the peripheral nervous system. When a sense dimension in TCM is associated with an organ and a phase, this reflects sensory experience rather than the physiologic transmission of stimuli. Prior to the discovery of the tubercular bacterium, the physiologically based term for the disease tuberculosis was consumption, a term based in sensory experience that accurately noted that the patient's physically wasted state was suggestive of being consumed by the disease.

Therapeutic practices designed to maintain existential robustness within the sense dimension of Touch will be introduced. Among these is drumming. If we had not understood that the call and response of successive drumbeats linked percussion with Touch, we might have classified drumming with hearing. Hearing-touch synesthesia (involvement of the Kidneys in TCM) is supported by a series of experiments reported in the journal *Nature* where the act of listening was shown to involve not only the ears but also the sense of Touch. In addition, sensations of touch were found to enhance what was auditorily perceived.[2]

Tuberculosis and Terrain Theory

In June 2012 coordinated research from the Human Microbiome Project Consortium organized by the National Institutes of Health (NIH) was released.

According to the stunning finding, two hundred scientists at eighty institutions sequenced the genetic material of bacteria taken from two hundred and fifty healthy people. More strains than they had ever imagined were discovered—as many as a thousand bacterial strains on each person. And each person's collection of microbes was unique. To the scientists' surprise they also found genetic signatures of pathological bacteria lurking in everyone's microbiome. But instead of making people ill or even infectious, these disease-causing microbes peacefully coexist with their neighbors.[3]

The "one germ, one disease" theory was promulgated by Louis Pasteur and others such as German scientist Robert Koch, a rival of Louis Pasteur often credited with having isolated the tuberculosis bacterium. Koch won the Nobel Prize for his work in 1905, but despite his impressive credentials he was exposed as an unscrupulous huckster by none other than the creator of Sherlock Holmes, physician-author Arthur Conan Doyle. He eventually was forced to divulge the embarrassing truth that his secret tubercular countermeasure was just a diluted glycerin extract of the tubercle bacillus itself.

Germ theory has long dominated allopathic medicine and been considered science-based, whereas terrain theory has been denigrated as relying on magical thinking. The Microbiome Project Consortium's findings, however, vindicate the terrain theory introduced by Claude Bernard (1813–1878) and further validated by Antoine Bechamp (1816–1908). Another rival of Pasteur, renowned as the father of pathology, Bechamp put an end to the theory of spontaneous generation. He also proposed that microzymas, not cells, are living entities within the body that coalesce to form blood clots and bacteria. His theory of zymotic disease posited that microzymas assume various forms depending upon the condition of the host: In a diseased body microzymas morph into pathological bacteria and viruses, whereas in a healthy body microzymas form healthy cells. When a plant or animal dies, the microzymas persist in living.

Bechamp maintained that the terrain, or internal environment, determines our state of health. When the body functions well it is in constant pursuit of homeostasis; immunity and the process of detoxification are then optimal. Such a healthy terrain is able to handle any pathogenic microorganisms it confronts. It is claimed that on his deathbed Pasteur himself came to agree with Bernard and repudiated the germ theory permanently affixed to his name.

The Human Microbiome Project Consortium's research indicates that an entire ecosystem of bacteria is symbiotically active within the body. Though long known by holistic practitioners and adepts of Bechamp, the concept is shocking to contemporary physicians: "This is a whole new way of looking at human biology and human disease," says Dr. Phillip Tarr, a researcher and professor of pediatrics at the Washington University School of Medicine. "It's awe-inspiring and it also offers incredible new opportunities."[4] Conceivably one day the tables will turn and it will be germ theory rather than terrain theory that is held up as an example of magical thinking.

One of the many bacilli residing within the human biome is *Mycobacterium tuberculosis*. Homeopaths perceive that tuberculosis is something other than an evil-intending scourge compressed into a bacillus in need of eradication. The bacillus has been with and within us at least as far back as the time of the Egyptian pharaohs, mostly slumbering within our biome, yet its virulence upon arousal has a purpose, which is to shout out an unmistakable and impossible-to-ignore command: "Our species should at once reestablish synchronic relations among its members! The foolishness of subjecting members of the human race to constricted freedom—impoverished existence amidst poverty, filth, and squalor—is intolerable! Convert the toxic intimacy of slum congestion into hygienic, touch-amenable housing and I, the tuberculin bacillus, will desist and return to my slumber."

Though examples abound, an alarming example of the culpability of congestion and poverty is the upsurge of tuberculosis is India, where more cases are found than in any other country—an estimated 2.3 million new cases each year. Many of these cases are found in horrifically engineered urban slums, such as those in Greater Mumbai, where more than nine million people, an estimated 41 percent of the population, live in poverty in 2023, with a dearth of windows and electricity.[5] Throughout India, 17.4 percent live in urban slums under those same conditions.[6]

A good source on Mumbai's tuberculosis and disease-resistant tuberculosis (DRT) problem is Vidya Krishnan's book, *Phantom Plague: How Tuberculosis Shaped History.*

With regard to tubercular infectivity, what can be offered to replace germ theory's misguided supposition that person-to-person transmission of *Mycobacterium tuberculosis* alone causes the disease? The answer is:

- Poverty and malnutrition that disharmonize terrain
- Proximity to biome-agitating human by-products, such as the toxic phlegm and sputum of individuals with overburdened immune systems
- Group "resonance," the "toxic touch" of ill and fearful people abiding in close quarters (the consciousness of people gathered in groups differing radically from that of the same individuals stationed apart)

The miasmatic influence of a disease can be acquired in several ways:

- Having in one's own lifetime been sickened by the disease
- Having inherited the influence of a disease, meaning it has

traversed one or more generations to energetically gain tenancy in
an individual

- Having acquired it through vaccination, meaning pharmaceutical
intervention aimed at suppressing the disease's symptoms

Earlier we learned that the tubercular miasm was not one of
Hahnemann's original three miasms. Henny Heudens-Mast explains
why: The tubercular miasm was not prominent in Hahnemann's time
because "most patients who contracted tuberculosis often died young or
did not marry or produce children, and therefore did not pass on the
disease in a miasm."[7]

The primary effects of the disease often go unnoticed early on.
Encyclopedia Britannica describes the disease's course as follows:

> The tubercle bacillus is a small, rod-shaped bacterium that is
> extremely hardy; it can survive for months in a state of dryness and
> can also resist the action of mild disinfectants. Infection spreads
> primarily by the respiratory route directly from an infected per-
> son who discharges live bacilli into the air. Minute droplets ejected
> by sneezing, coughing, and even talking can contain hundreds of
> tubercle bacilli that may be inhaled by a healthy person. There the
> bacilli become trapped in the tissues of the body, are surrounded by
> immune cells, and finally are sealed up in hard, nodular tubercles. A
> tubercle usually consists of a centre of dead cells and tissues, cheese-
> like (caseous) in appearance, in which can be found many bacilli.
> This centre is surrounded by radially arranged phagocytic (scaven-
> ger) cells and a periphery containing connective tissue cells. The
> tubercle thus forms as a result of the body's defensive reaction to
> the bacilli. Individual tubercles are microscopic in size, but most of
> the visible manifestations of tuberculosis, from barely visible nodules
> to large tuberculous masses, are conglomerations of tubercles.[8]

The physiological basis for the existential theme of restricted freedom mentioned earlier is now suggested: Bacilli covered by tough
tissue compose the disease's characteristic respiration-impeding

tubercle. The tubercle's lung-capacity-reducing presence makes the patient yearn to breathe free and in other ways seek freedom as well. This is expressed in the tubercular miasm's restless, readily bored, fulfillment-seeking features.

Tuberculosis's association with poverty has a parallel in homeopathic theory. Earlier we learned of this miasm's comorbidity with the oldest miasm, the psora (and also the syphilitic miasm), for which reason it was originally referred to as a pseudo-psora, in regard to which we recall that psora's existential concern with poverty and dearth.

FIRE PHASE AND
TRADITIONAL CHINESE MEDICINE

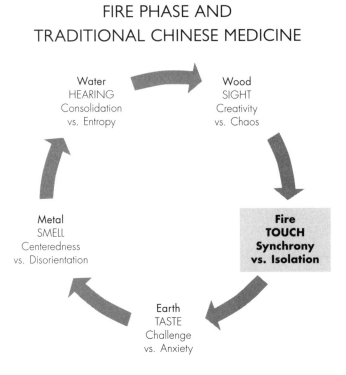

Water
HEARING
Consolidation
vs. Entropy

Wood
SIGHT
Creativity
vs. Chaos

Fire
TOUCH
Synchrony
vs. Isolation

Metal
SMELL
Centeredness
vs. Disorientation

Earth
TASTE
Challenge
vs. Anxiety

In TCM the Heart is viewed as the master of blood and its channels. Since it also houses the spirit or mind it is more accurate to refer to this organ as the Heart/Mind. The Heart and its paired organ, the Small Intestine, belong to the phase (or element) of Fire. Fire generates fever, heat, redness, and agitation when it is excessive. Pallor, coldness, or aversion to cold appear when it is deficient. Though pertaining to the phase of Water, the Kidneys also possess an accessory Fire function, likened to a pilot light for the totality of the body's chi (vital energy).

Although the Heart is the master of blood, in TCM two other organs provide important related functions: The Liver is the storehouse of blood and contributes to blood's smooth distribution, and the Spleen maintains blood in its correct pathways. Problems such as hypertension or painful menses may involve the Heart, Liver, Spleen, and/or Kidneys.

Symptoms of Heart disharmonies in TCM include weak or irregular pulse, coldness, cyanosis (skin discoloration due to deficient blood oxygenation), insomnia, anxiety, emotional instability, depression, agitation, and various manias. Biomedical diagnoses could include arrhythmia, angina pectoris, arteriosclerosis, anemia, hypertension, edema, epilepsy, stroke sequelae, neurosis, depression, bipolar disorder, and psychosis.

TCM's nomenclature associating the Fire phase with blood circulation and the Heart indicates how tuberculosis (consumption) manifests heart and circulation pathology.

In New England, more than two centuries after the hysteria of the witch trials, there was another kind of panic. Consumption claimed 2 percent of New England's population—the lives of entire families in Rhode Island, Connecticut, Vermont, and other parts of the northeast—between 1786, when health officials first began recording mortality rates, and 1800. The death toll was horrific and the slow, agonizing death equally so. Consumptives became emaciated, they coughed blood, and their skin turned pale and ashen. Something seemed to be sucking the life out of the victims, and the belief arose that the deceased were rising up out of the grave to suck the life out of their surviving relatives. See Vidya Krishnan's chapter on "The Grave of Mercy Brown," a suspected vampire of that era.[9]

SYNCHRONY VS. ISOLATION

Synchrony manifests everywhere. Electrons act in concert as coupled oscillators. In the seventeenth century physicist Christiaan Huygens, inventor of the pendulum clock, observed that two pendulums suspended from a single beam will sometimes adjust to swing consistently in opposite directions. Without colliding with one another a flock of birds on the wing will in unison suddenly shift direction. Thousands of fireflies can flash in unison. Social trends and mass hysteria spontaneously arise.

Alpha waves fire in synchronicity across billions of neurons in the brain, where their combined electrical signals oscillate in the frequency of 8 to 12 hertz. When manipulated in the course of neurofeedback therapy, alpha waves filter out distracting sensory information. The "all-at-onceness" of synchronistic brain waves is reflected in another tubercular feature spoken of in homeopathy texts as a "desire to be magnetized." The tubercular miasm's most prominent metal remedy, Phosphorus, strongly exhibits this affinity for connection along with a closely related liability, an excessive permeability of boundaries.

We can expand upon Carl Jung's notion of synchronicity when circumstances strike us as meaningfully related despite absent causal connection. Rather than causal, two unexpectedly alike or identical events are related through identity. Pertaining to an energetic field that we as perceivers are normally privy to encounter one element at a time, my conjecture is that synchronic events are actually one and the same phenomenon. When activities within the pertaining field increase, what Rupert Sheldrake termed "morphic resonance"—a process whereby systems or structures of activity inherit a memory from previous similar systems—occurs as inherited collective memory. Experience of synchronic events then tends to surge. I can offer some recent examples:

- Years back I blogged about successfully treating a patient with non-Hodgkin's lymphoma. My method involved performing moxibustion (the burning of an herb, *Artemisia vulgaris*) on an anticancer acupuncture point, Pee Gun (root of tumor), taught to me by a great teacher, James Tin Yao So. For seven years I had not been called on to perform this treatment, nor during all this time had I received a single response to my blog. Yesterday afternoon, seven years later, I was asked to provide this treatment for a client with cancer. Later that evening, "out of the blue," from an acupuncturist in Italy I received my very first response to the cancer moxibustion blog. It was from an acupuncturist seeking more information about how to treat the Pee Gun point. Had my treatment reverberated across the Atlantic Ocean?

- This past week, while taking the case of a woman frantic about changing her life to accommodate artistic and spiritual yearnings, I experienced a strong sense of déjà vu. I soon realized the "having experienced this before" feeling was not déjà vu but actual. A few weeks earlier I had had precisely the same conversation with another woman client. Fancying that these women might be psychic twins, I looked up the prior client in my files and discovered that they were of exactly the same age. A remedy I had prescribed for the earlier client made from the gemstone black opal now appeared correct for my current client. When I showed her an image of the black opal gem, she gasped. Its blue-black, galaxy-like appearance was exactly what she had been creating in her own current art (images later emailed confirmed this was true).

- After taking the case of a guilt-ridden client, I decided that the remedy Cobaltum (described in the psora chapter) was correct for him. In the course of explaining the remedy and its theme of feeling like a criminal while everyone knew it, I related the story of General Motors Corporation initially trying to hide an engineering problem in its Cobalt model; eventually the company was outed and forced to recall thousands of its foolishly named (in German it means goblin or evil spirit) automobiles. Suddenly his eyes widened. Two days earlier his own car, he told me, had been rear-ended by a Chevy Cobalt.

The emerging science of synchrony described by Steven Strogatz in his book *Sync: The Emerging Science of Spontaneous Order* suggests that the central mechanism operating within living things is a biological clock. Keeping time to a circadian rhythm or some such pattern, biological activity unfolds. Rather than according to its organs and physiology, we might better define an organism as a network of biological clocks having evolved to behave in synchrony with one another. A philosophical term suggestive of synchrony and used in medieval philosophy is *entelechy:* the realization of potential that guides the development and functioning of an organism or other organized system. Entelechy denotes or accounts for how living things cluster purposively in time: why cells form themselves into tissue, bison run in a herd, fish swim in a school, or human beings seek community. The outbreak of an unexpected "insistence" on integrity within an organic system—spontaneous healing—we term super-synchrony.[10]

Synchrony is typically at play when bonding among individuals and communion with the greater wholes of community, ecosystem, and spiritual domain is at issue. It operates in group identification, falling in love, merging into the flow of traffic in a rotary, and joining in applause with others even when one has not appreciated a performance. As noted when Touch was discussed earlier, not all synchrony denotes health. Cancer cells cluster synchronously into a tumor. Crowds can turn riotous.

If synchrony is the positive pole of the synchrony-isolation axis, then isolation—being out of touch, out of step, not in rhythm, and unable to act for a common purpose—is the negative pole. Isolation underlies numerous psychological ills that TCM classifies as ailments of the Heart. Reconnecting the individual to relationships that both honor and exceed the self is then required.

From a biomedical perspective, as an extension of the heart the three coronary arteries are synchronically aligned. If the heart's supply of blood and oxygen is reduced, the heart responds to that call by down-regulating its own energy needs. If the progress of arterial blockage in one artery does not occur too quickly, the communicating branches compensate by gradually widening.

A slightly variable heartbeat is actually healthier than one steady as a metronome. An unvarying rhythm represents rigidity, tension, and an overly circumscribed response to stress. The alignment of emotions, cardiovascular reactions, and brain states is evident in mothers and their infants, in marital partners arguing, and within committees.

Heart/mind synchrony is found in the function of mirror neurons. These neurons fire not only when an individual performs a task but when the individual observes another person performing the task. Social bonding and rapport with one another are thus neurologically ordained. That we are hardwired for interconnectivity is famously endorsed by the Elizabethan-era writer John Donne, who wrote:

> No man is an island, entire of itself; every man is a piece of the continent, a part of the main; if a clod be washed away by the sea, Europe is the less, as well as if a promontory were, as well as if a manor of thy friend's or of thine own were; any man's death diminishes me, because I am involved in mankind, and therefore never send to know for whom the bell tolls; it tolls for thee.[11]

The Tubercular Miasm's Existential Themes

- Basic right to hygienic existence devoid of poverty, squalor, and filth
- Synchrony, not isolation; taking relationships to heart
- Return to the source
- Having it all at once; restlessness
- One must breathe and live free
- Fulfillment in life

TREATMENTS AND EXPECTATIONS

Remedies manifesting subcategories of *Am I alone in life or do I act in synchrony with nature and with others?*

Aconitum napellus	Mancinella
Apis mellifica	Phosphorus
Arsenicum album	Rhus radicans
Belladonna	Tarentula hispanica
Calcarea phosphorica	Tuberculinum Koch

Aconitum napellus
In touch with my death

Restlessness	**Forethought of death**
Suddenness/shock	**Dry, burning heat**

The extreme restlessness and sudden onset of symptoms of the Aconitum napellus state pegs it as a tubercular remedy. A person needing this remedy made from monkswood has had a sudden and frightening taste of death, after which symptoms come on rapidly. Acute, violent, and painful, they appear suddenly, remaining for a short while, like a big storm that quickly blows over. A patient's nerves are excited and she experiences emotional and nervous tension for which reason the mind is affected. She becomes frantic, screams, groans, gnaws the fist, bites the nails, wants to die. Fear accompanies her most trivial ailments. Heart and arterial circulation is affected, with congestion to the head (often apoplectic) and chest. Aconitum is a remedy for acute inflammation and congestion. Sensations of burning, numbness, tingling, prickling, or crawling are marked. Body parts feel large or deformed. There is external soreness, with internal heaviness, sudden loss of strength, and possible collapse.

The remedy state includes complaints caused by exposure to cold, dry weather, especially respiratory affections. Constantine Hering's description of Aconitum napellus noted:

- Fear of ghosts; fear of loss of reason; apprehensive of the future
- Fear of approaching death; predicts the day of death
- Inconsolable anxiety; piteous wailing; reproaches others for mere trifles; peevish, impatient; pusillanimous
- Anxious, restless, agonized tossing about
- Oversensitive, cannot bear light or noise; buzzing in the ears; will not be touched or uncovered
- Mood is peevish, irritable, malicious or sad, despondent
- After a fright, afraid in the dark
- After fright with vexation or anger, heat, congestion, threatened abortion; ailments from fright following later
- Ailments from anger or from chagrin; in a child, spells of rage
- Imagines some part of the body is deformed, thinks from the stomach
- Fear of approaching death; predicts the day[12]

This is a major remedy for panic disorder such as can arise long after an initial shock. Women who have experienced exhausting and painful childbirth are often sent home from the hospital scant days after delivery. Once home, many immediately must resume cooking, caretaking, and managing the household. Months later, after a routine has been established and when one might think the new mother can finally breathe more easily, a panic disorder sets in. *Remember me?* the psyche is chiding. *We almost died! This business is not yet settled!* Aconite should then be given.

Apis mellifica

Shall I be fruitful or shall I multiply?

Restlessness	Family orientation
Aggravation from heat	Creativity vs. procreativity
Shock	Stinging pain

This remedy's restlessness and affinity for reproduction's return-to-the-source theme places it in the tubercular category. Made from honeybee venom (actually from crushed, angry honeybees), the Apis mellifica remedy mirrors the natural history of the bee, a creature hell-bent on the tasks of work and reproduction. Apis mellifica treats edema in cases in which there is a strong underlying conflict between work and reproduction, between being fruitful and multiplying. The patient seeks synchrony among, and benefit for, current family members, but this choice is frequently a conflicted one, and if unresolved, the conflict promotes pathology. Recent bereavement, the need to care for an ill parent, or a financial setback can serve as a shock that initiates an Apis mellifica state. In addition to edema, physical symptoms of Apis mellifica may include urticaria (hives), cystic ovaries, hardening of the skin, restlessness, shortness of breath, stinging pains, and aggravation from heat.

As with a bee sting, the Apis mellifica picture's edema is the consequence of an inflammatory reaction. What is in Apis mellifica that connects the phenomenon of inflammation with problematic fertility? The answer appears to be an inflammatory enzyme that facilitates the spread of fluids, hyaluronidase, which not so coincidentally is present within both bee venom and the acrosome (or the "warhead" of human sperm that releases egg-penetrating enzymes). Contact with hyaluronidase, in fact, is what breaches the ovum's membrane and gains the sperm's entrance to the egg. The radical disjunct (see below) here is that the desire to reproduce promotes the need to set limits on family size.

Modeling Constitutional Polarities; Radical Disjunct

Radical disjunct is a useful approach for identifying and modeling key contributions or paradoxes within constitutional remedy states. Suggestive of the ego defense mechanism Sigmund Freud designated as a reaction formation, a radical disjunct occurs when provision of the normal fulfillment of a need not only fails to quench the need but makes it worse. Consider an individual who fears being close to dirt. His vigilant pursuit of cleanliness and passion to eradicate filth brings him ever closer to dirt's proximity. Fear of contacting dirt creates more contact with dirt. This self-reinforcing feedback loop perpetuates itself. As opposed to reaction formation, which describes behavior, the radical disjunct's capacity to encompass physical symptomatology sustains an imbalance or a chronic illness. Sense-dimensional analysis illuminates how a radical disjunct promotes chronic illness.

Identification of the radical disjunct is central to deconstructing complex and often paradoxical descriptions of homeopathic remedies. For example, the radical disjunct of the homeopathic remedy Nux vomica lies in its indication for someone who, though irritable, impatient, controlling, and in constant battle mode, claims that all he wants is a little peace. He has the excessive energy of a multitasker but complains of exhaustion. Though logically the two extremes ought to cancel one another out, they fail to do so.

A radical disjunct can arise iatrogenically. For example, a medication for depression heightens the risk for suicide; a medication to treat softening of the bones and susceptibility to fracture causes bones to become brittle. Failure to resolve an underlying issue is generally the cause.

Arsenicum album

Is my circle of love secure?

No margin for error	Inner burning/outer chill
Anxiety	Restlessness
Death is approaching	Prostration

What makes Arsenicum album tubercular (it also fits other miasmatic classifications) is its restlessness and feeling of isolation. When an individual is poisoned with non-homeopathic arsenic, the experience is a presentiment of death. Accordingly time is short; affairs must be in order and loved ones safeguarded. The remedy state thus manifests great restlessness, anxiety, melancholy, concern for reserves of money and aging, loneliness, and a sense of being unable to find rest anywhere, of wanting to move from bed to bed. The mindset also includes suicidality, inclination to self-mutilation; insomnia but also awakening from pain, especially after midnight. Arsenicum album will also be discussed in the next chapter as a psoric remedy.

Belladonna

Do I belong in this world or in another?

Intense/throbbing	Desire to strike
Hallucination (animals, insects)	Rush of blood to head
Delirium/joy	Heat/redness/burning restlessness

Belladonna (deadly nightshade) is of great value in cases of hysteria. This includes nighttime terrors, oversensitivity, wild delirium, furious rages, fits of laughter, teeth-grinding, fear of dogs, hallucinations, and a sense that one is dreaming while wide awake.

In keeping with the tubercular miasm, emotions flare with sudden and brief intensity. Phobias are present, such as fear of the cutting of hair, of the head becoming wet, of exposure to the sun or wind, or of being shaken. The condition reflects the excessive imagination, sensitivities, and fears native to childhood. Physical symptoms include congestion and pulsation in the head and headaches. The radical disjunct here is that investment in freedom of the imagination promotes its opposite—isolation within a self-contained world.

Belladonna manifests TCM's understanding of the uprooted ethereal soul. As opposed to the corporeal soul that inhabits the Lungs and is mortal, the ethereal soul inhabits the Liver. Rather than perishing following death, it returns to its source in the collective unconscious. Overactivity of the ethereal soul accounts for sleeplessness and the night terrors of a child needing Belladonna. Children are more prone than adults to fall into this state, with the ethereal soul intruding more easily into their consciousness.

Calcarea phosphorica

Shall I expand or constrain my horizons?

Restless/inattentive	Cannot bear bad news
Boredom/love of travel	Bones, joints, teeth
Growth spurts	Worse from cold and wind

Calcarea phosphorica's restlessness and quickness to boredom place it in the tubercular miasm. The physical presentation reflects the nutrition of bones and glands. Bones become soft, thin, and brittle, but they also will ossify if in the wake of a fracture the bones heal poorly. Glands are swollen. Patients, especially children, are delicate, tall, and thin or scrawny, with brownish or discolored skin. They tend to emaciation and anemia following acute illness. Other features of the remedy state include trembling or trembling hands and coldness or soreness in spots such as the top of the head, eyeballs, and tip of the nose and fingers.

The remedy is prominent in a peculiar rubric: Home, desire to go, and when there, to go out again. This is a radical disjunct: The Calc phosphorica individual seeks protection and security from the company of others. Yet attainment of companionship, rather than satisfying her need for security prompts something opposite: desire for freedom and the leeway to explore possibilities outside the bounds of security. Calcarea phosphorica, which is a major mineral component of the bones, comes up strongly during growth spurts in teenagers. It is then as if their bones are confused on this issue. It is as if they say to themselves: *I am the skel-*

eton and everything hangs on me. But it seems that now the body's need to develop demands that I suspend my body-stabilizing mission.

The remedy comes into play when teeth (that are also bone) develop slowly, are soft, or have rapid decay. The issue is not trivial, for in someone needing this remedy, problems with cognition can appear. Also, the Calcarea phosphorica individual cannot bear hearing bad news. Not that anyone likes hearing bad news, but due to immaturity and insecurity the Calcarea phosphorica person handles this especially poorly. Her body may communicate this somatically by causing formication (a skin-crawling sensation) and numbness as a result.

Mancinella

Dark thoughts possess me

> Having lost control of my thoughts, I am going mad
> Evil is approaching; the future is horrible
> Delirium; thoughts instantly vanish
> Diminished intellect; depression
> Vivacity and sexual erethism (easily excited)
> Burning, biting, smarting pains
> Choking sensation in throat

Though typically presenting in someone older than a child, much as with Belladonna, Mancinella represents and addresses the mental hazards of youth, a time when exposure to a violent event or frightening spectacle leaves an indelible impression. Featuring delirium, terror of the future, and fear of insanity, Mancinella manifests isolation triumphing over synchrony. By dint of the suddenness of reactions, such as constriction of the throat and esophagus and the immediately vanishing thoughts, Mancinella is classified a tubercular remedy. In keeping with the sense dimension of Touch, its burning sensations align with TCM's Fire phase. The doorway to Mancinella is the experience of having witnessed something frightening. Feeling haunted and expecting something horrible to happen afterward is not surprising. On an ominous note, in recent years I have had to prescribe the remedy more and more often. Hopefully this trend will abate.

Phosphorus

The spark of life

Restless/spaced out	Clairvoyance
Great return	Grief
Charismatic	Wherever the inorganic
Excessively permeable	becomes organic
boundaries	

Phosphorus is the element most closely associated with the tubercular miasm. It has a glow that obscures its source, making it difficult to see where the substance begins and ends. Consistent with this feature, Phosphorus individuals have trouble setting boundaries, expressed in their tendency to hemorrhage (the blood does not remain within the capillaries), to connect too readily with strangers, and to manifest spaciness and scattered thinking. Key rubrics in which Phosphorus is prominent relate to oversensitivity to impressions, an artistic temperament, reactivity to thunderstorms, vibrancy, an appealing nature, and having a flair for color.

Phosphorus individuals are susceptible to respiratory problems, hypoglycemia, prostration, inflammation, and degeneration of the mucous membranes of the stomach, bowels, and nerves. The remedy state reflects or promotes disorganization of the blood, causing fatty degeneration of blood vessels and every tissue and organ of the body.

Phosphorus patients exhibit anxiety, a counterbalancing reaction to having taken too much in. Grief affects them greatly. An understanding of the biochemical role of phosphorus illuminates this feature: Along with hydrogen, oxygen, nitrogen, and carbon, phosphorus is one of only five elements constituting DNA, the genetic material of all living organisms. It is a key component of adenosine diphosphate (ADP), an ester of adenosine that is converted to adenosine triphosphate (ATP) for the storage of energy and is the basic energy unit of aerobic metabolism. Phosphorylation, the introduction of a phosphate group into a molecule (the first stage in a reaction that can produce ATP), enables inert organic compounds to become biochemically active. Phosphorus is also required in the formation of bones and teeth.

Phosphorus, which can be combustible, is imbued with the spark of life. Its presence in chemical reactions prompts subtle events, allowing inert matter to quicken. Without phosphorus, organic life cannot code or respire; muscles do not twitch. With phosphorus, heavily mineralized substances become tissue; teeth and bones acquire a living core. As phosphorus is an incredibly precious resource, a looming global phosphorus shortage aggravated by soil erosion is ominous. This metal's depletion from agricultural systems will delimit future food and feed production.

In keeping with the themes of Fire and Touch, Phosphorus's challenge is to maintain proximity to the source of creation; its anxiety is to avoid becoming apprehensive or frightened during the encounter.

Rhus radicans

Structure versus freedom

Restless/better from movement	Ritualistic
Stiff joints/back	Itching
"Rusty gate"	Dwells on the past

Rhus radicans, derived from the poison ivy plant, is similar to Calcarea phosphorica for its extreme restlessness.* Patients are often itchy and drawn to a routine to the point of becoming superstitious. The mindset pertaining to this challenge concerns being tightly contained within a structure from which one must then also burst free. This creates a situation in which sudden movement is destabilizing. The remedy state is closely related to golf, in which the swing of the club demands exact repeatability (the need to reach varying distances is met by switching clubs as opposed to altering the swing), and one's adversary is only oneself. Golfers are especially prone to back pain, often arthritic, for which Rhus radicans is a key remedy.

It is not unusual for cold and damp to be found in combination. Individuals in need of Rhus radicans suffer from a "rusty gate"

---

*Rhus radicans has long been incorrectly termed Rhus toxicodendron, which is derived from poison oak.

syndrome in that they experience severe stiffness of the joints that is made worse by the cold or dampness and ameliorated by stretching and movement.

Though not stuck in the past (as we shall see in the sycosis miasm), Rhus radicans individuals find themselves hearkening back to unhappy events from the past. They do so repetitiously, as if adhering to a script.

Tarentula hispanica

Dancing to the beat of my own drum

Unrequited love	Reactive to music
Hurries others	Twitching, ticks
Destructive/cunning	Wants to be noticed
Quickness/jumping	Feels suffocated

Tarentula hispanica is tubercular by way of the respiratory problem, a tendency for the individual to feel she is suffocating, incredible restlessness, and a quality that is the opposite of synchrony: dysrhythmia. The individual needing this remedy moves with incredible quickness but disjointedly, manifesting the consciousness and movements of at least five different species of spider, summarized by the name *Tarentula hispanica*. Morbid synchrony here manifests as a disordered rhythm in the electrical activity of the heart; abnormal, rapid, rhythmic movements of the body; an aversion to being touched; palpitations; hyperactivity; impulsiveness; restlessness; and a need to hurry other people. The symptoms present as despair, melancholy, wildness, cunning, and incontinence.

A gateway to the remedy state is unrequited love in compensation for which the hyper behavior screams, "You must take notice of me," which by way of radical disjunct prompts a disengagement response from others. Such individuals are touch avoidant and cannot bear a reprimand. Their relationships lack a normal rhythm, alternating between dependency and possessiveness and shifting rapidly from flight to fight. This individual will have a great affinity for percussive music, music in general, dancing, horseback riding, and sexual activity.

Tuberculinum Koch

I must breathe freely

An anti-squalor "sermon"	Respiratory ailments
Restless/bored	Craves freedom
Unfulfilled/romantic	Destructive
Love for the outdoors	

Here once again is the nosode (remedy derived from an infectious disease product) of the tubercular miasm discussed at length at the beginning of this chapter. We recall the "sermon" the remedy preaches: that synchronic relations among humans benefit everyone; that unless we cease to countenance poverty, squalor, and malnutrition, the scourge of tuberculosis will regularly visit and ravage our terrain.

By way of reviewing its effects that form a template for other remedies in the tubercular miasm, its prime domain is the mind, lungs, head, occiput, glands, and larynx. Its symptoms constantly change. They begin suddenly, cease suddenly, or are obscure and difficult to quell even with a well-selected remedy. The tubercular miasm state reflects or promotes weakness and emaciation (though with good appetite). The patient takes cold easily after the slightest exposure and soon develops diarrhea. Such individuals are susceptible to illness due to weather change. Illness relapse is common. Exhaustion and lowered vitality tend to increase. Rapid breakdown is seen. The state is adapted to light-complexioned, narrow-chested subjects; mentally deficient children; individuals prone to seizures; and nervous, weak, and tremulous people.

In addition to acupuncture, homeopathy, and biomedicine, various personal therapeutic practices promote existential robustness within the sense dimension of Touch.

Touch Dimension Health Promotion Practices

- Devotional practices
- Massage
- Philanthropy
- Yoga, Reiki
- Reverence for origins
- Poetry
- Drumming, dance, song
- Spiritual involvement

2

Is my presence in the world sustainable?

Psoric Miasm • Taste • Earth Phase •
Worry • Spleen–Stomach

We enter this world naked and vulnerable. Will we be taken care of? Protected? Nourished? Loved? These questions lie at the heart of what I have termed the sense dimension of Taste and underlie inborn susceptibility to the psoric miasm. As discussed earlier, in terms of the screwdriver of anxiety of the Inborn Toolkit, overcoming challenges related to biting off more than we can chew also figures into the psoric miasm.

THE PSORIC MIASM AND THE SENSE DIMENSION OF TASTE

Samuel Hahnemann maintained that nonvenereal chronic diseases, comprising the majority of chronic diseases, such as skin diseases, most mental ailments (other than those of a syphilitic origin), allergies, varicose veins, hemorrhoids, and many dysfunctional diseases of organs and systems, are psoric in origin. Indicating a "primordial itch," the word's origin is Greek. A similar word from Hebrew, *tsorat,* refers to a groove or stigma. According to homeopathy's founder, psora is the most ancient and insidious miasm. It is derived from prior skin eruptions such as

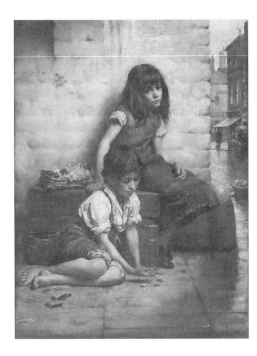

Waifs, a painting by
Thomas Kennington

scabies, leprosy, and psoriasis contracted during a patient's childhood or transmitted as an ancestral legacy. According to Hahnemann, suppression of these conditions through the use of balms, emollients, or other lotions lies at the root cause of psora.

Invoking morality-inflected principles, renowned Hahnemann disciple James Tyler Kent expanded the theory by proposing psora as the foundation of all other illness. Given a hypothetical absence of psora, Kent maintained mankind would live in the Garden of Eden in a pure and illness-free state. Psora is equated with man's fall from original grace into sinfulness. From this notion it was but a small step for Kent to position psora as also the foundation of the sexual miasms, as he did later.

In the wake of Kent's influence within homeopathic practice the list of remedies associated with psora came to expand so greatly that the miasm's principal psychological theme, all-encompassing as it might be, grew clouded. By way of response this book's alternative—hopefully clarifying—model of psora is proposed. A number of psoric remedies prominent in the treatment of skin conditions guide us through psora's subcategory themes, the broad perspective of which is, *I am somehow not okay in the world,* and the narrow perspective of which is a concern that *The sustaining of my material existence is in doubt.* The following discussion of what I have termed the sense dimension of Taste elaborates on this point.

The Sense Dimension of Taste

Wuxing phase: Earth
Emotion: Worry
Organ: Spleen-Stomach (metabolism)
Theme: Challenge vs. anxiety

As the root word of *sapience* (wisdom, knowledge) is the Latin *sapere* (to taste), the sense dimension of Taste denotes contemplation and thought. The sense of taste underlies our ability to make distinctions. When Adam and Eve tasted the apple they were enabled to distinguish between good and evil. Research evidence supports the idea that the tongue contains numerous flavor receptors. All parts of the tongue's surface, in fact, can detect every flavor: fifty to one hundred receptors exist for each of the basic tastes, which allows for considerable variation in individual taste. The tongue's chemical receptors delineate not only sweet, salty, sour, and bitter, but also *umami* (from the Japanese), a savory flavor associated with meats, some cheeses, and mushrooms. Umami receptors are stimulated by monosodium glutamate, a taste-enhancing food additive. In addition to these five tastes, the tongue may have chemical receptors for fat.

Synthesizing taste, smell, and touch (texture and temperature) creates flavor, to which memory contributes a flavoring perception. Smell serves to amplify flavor identification. A thousand smells but only a handful of tastes can be identified, explaining why disturbances in flavor perception are mostly due to sense-of-smell-related disorders. Dysfunction in the taste component of flavor perception can be due to dryness of the mouth, oral infection, certain medications, radiation injury, burns, nutritional deficiencies, Bell's palsy, and dentures. Aging, since it can reduce the acuity of both taste and smell, is an additional risk factor.

EARTH PHASE AND
TRADITIONAL CHINESE MEDICINE

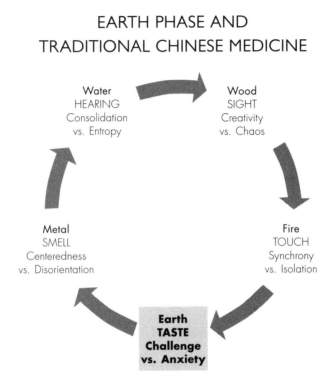

The Spleen

In Traditional Chinese Medicine the Spleen, due to its responsibility for separating the pure from the impure and then transporting the resulting products appropriately throughout the body, holds dominion over the transformation of food and drink. Chi and blood thus nourish the muscles, for which reason the Spleen is said to rule the muscles and limbs. Its failure to do so produces fatigue and muscular atrophy.

The Spleen governs the blood. This prevents hemorrhages as the blood is sequestered in its proper channels. Spleen *yang* (its active, energetic aspect) is also thought to hold organs in position, preventing prolapses. The Spleen's transforming and transporting functions pertain to the production and movement of all fluids in the body. Thus, its fluid functions support and overlap those of the Kidneys. Biomedically speaking, TCM's Spleen incorporates the functions of the pancreas while also holding responsibility for the storage of cellular energy, meaning cellular respiration, which produces carriers of chemical energy within cells. Considered part of the Spleen within ancient Chinese medicine, the pancreas produces insulin to regulate blood sugar as well as digestive enzymes.

The Spleen and its paired organ, the Stomach, pertain to the phase of Earth. Within Wuxing, Earth connotes stability, nurturance, and compassion, such as in the archetype of an earth mother. The season it relates to within the Table of Correspondences from which the Five Phases are drawn is a fifth season, late summer, which comes between summer and autumn.

The Spleen is the postnatal foundation of health. Its function extends to supplying the nutritive fractions that generate the chi and blood necessary to sustain life and nourish all the other organs. For this reason the Earth phase is held to occupy a central position in health and illness. Besides hemorrhages and prolapses, symptoms of Spleen disharmonies in TCM include edema, excess phlegm, cloudy urine, muscular atrophy, dizziness, seizures, fatigue, metabolic disorders, and a large number of digestive disorders. Lost or diminished sense of taste signals a disturbance of the Spleen.

TASTE DIMENSION CORE ISSUE: THE CHALLENGE-ANXIETY AXIS

Doubt concerning the sustaining of one's material existence in psora is expanded upon in our discussion of the sense dimension of Taste where a challenge-versus-anxiety conundrum is found to be central.

Substances taken into the mouth as food are effectively screened there for nutritive suitability. Toxicity, too, can be quickly gauged. Taste is thus the first arbiter of the life-or-death digestive distinctions encountered with every bite. A subtle and proper edge of anxiety attends this venturing forth of taste. Anxiety associated with taste in the act of eating is mirrored at another level by anxiety in the act of obtaining food. Whether during the uncertainties and hazards of hunting or with struggles through lean seasons, pursuit of sustenance is linked with primal anxiety. The anxiety of obtaining food is experienced by every infant, newly dependent on external sources of food.

Producing cellular energy presents such significant challenges to the body that it has invested in backup systems to provide coverage in the event of failure or overload. Mitochondria, cell organelles that generate energy for cells, produce chemical energy carriers—high-energy molecules such as adenosine triphosphate (ATP). Defects in ATP production may stem from abnormalities in nutrient uptake, in the Krebs cycle of aerobic reactions, in oxidative phosphorylation, or in errors of genetic signaling. Cumulative mitochondrial damage (as happens from chronic exposure to free radicals) contributes to fatigue, functional aging, and other symptoms consistent with Spleen chi deficiency.

An imperfect safety net, the anaerobic backup system is maintained to countenance the high challenges of aerobic metabolism. It provides an example of the challenge-anxiety axis operating at the level of cellular biochemistry. Given severe energy demands, or when mitochondria fail, cells fall back on anaerobic metabolic pathways so that high-energy molecules are generated. Though less efficient than aerobic metabolism, anaerobic metabolism allows us to survive, although just barely. The organs most adversely impacted by mitochondrial disorders are the higher energy users, including the brain, skeletal and cardiac muscle, sensory organs, and kidneys. Mitochondrial disorders are possibly at the root of chronic fatigue syndrome.

CHALLENGE VS. ANXIETY

Master Yunmen was asked, "What is most urgent for me?" The master answered, "The very *you* who is afraid that he doesn't know."[1]

With this answer the master points out that anxiety is rooted in fear of the unknown and that our constant challenge is its overcoming.

Challenge

Whether accepted or invited, the little brother of anxiety grows up into the big brother of challenge. The psychological, biological, and material will to obtain mastery over anxiety is exemplified in the hunt, whose fearsome challenge functions as a staging ground for entry into adulthood. As we sometimes bite off more than we can chew (and then must chew it over), grounds for challenge are also found in the process of eating.

Once the body accepts a challenge, its biological response is to cash in one or more units of fuel currency, namely, the molecule ATP. A recent discovery with regard to the ATP molecule supports the notion that challenge is directly and immediately associated with the mouth. In addition to providing the body with fuel, ATP performs the additional essential function of being a non-neuronal neurotransmitter conveying information regarding the sense perception of taste, as well as that of other senses. When released by non-neuronal cells like those found in the oral cavity, ATP triggers protective responses within the body that may build bone that is calculated to meet a challenge. The gut faces the challenge of transporting ingested materials, breaking them down into absorbable forms, extracting nutrients, and ridding the body of waste products. At every stage in the carefully gated process of transport—breakdown, assimilation, and rejection— the potential for costly error must be thwarted.

Anxiety

What the Wuxing calls worry, we refer to as anxiety. Anxiety that begins with taste makes itself known in the depths of the gut. The enteric nervous system is a brain within the lining of the gastrointestinal tract, extending from mid-esophagus to the anus. It has autonomous functions but is connected with the central nervous system by the vagus nerve. Relying on the same neurotransmitters as the cranial brain, the enteric nervous system controls local blood flow, directs propulsion along the digestive tract, and influences absorption. Under stress it can shut down the digestive system or signal it to empty by means of excretion or vomiting. It can also trigger an immune response, causing mast cells to release histamine in the lining of the small intestine and colon. The enteric nervous system samples the contents of the intestinal tract with chemoreceptors that react to acids, sugars, and amino acids. By chemically ascertaining anxiety of fight-or-flight situations, our brain in the gut is empowered to make key distinctions.

The body's ability to perform expulsion is a functional aspect of anxiety. A judgment is made within the dimension of taste that a pathogen, a nonviable fetus or a baby at full-term, a transplanted organ, a morsel of food lodged in the esophagus, or an ingested toxin can no longer be accommodated or assimilated. The body then mobilizes to repel or expel the substance by sneezing, coughing, gagging, vomiting, downshifting of bowel, or uterine motility.

In parallel with Hahnemann and Kent's understanding that psora covers the majority of medical conditions, we also find that more ailments reflect disharmony within the sense dimension of Taste than in any other sense dimension.

The Psoric Miasm's Existential Themes

- Anxious, not okay in the world
- What I have today is not enough for tomorrow
- Not safe, sheltered, or nourished
- Insecurity
- Anxiety vs. challenge
- Nurturance
- Competition vs. compliance

TREATMENTS AND EXPECTATIONS

Remedies manifesting subcategories of *Is my presence in the world sustainable?*

Aceticum acidum	Falco peregrinus
Arsenicum album	Kali bichromicum
Calcarea carbonica	Kali bromatum
Camphora	Lycopodium clavatum
Clematis recta	Mezereum
Cobaltum metallicum	Psorinum

Aceticum acidum
Disenfranchised

Anemic	Emaciation
Anxious for family, children	Worries about business affairs
"Borrows trouble"	Stupor
Abdominal complaints	Self-deprecating

Acticum acidum is an infrequently used remedy whose physical symptoms are more definite than its core issue. Its realm of action encompasses weakness, faintness, and swooning to the point of stupor, as well as muscular flaccidity, anemia, emaciation, edema, gastralgia, and dyspepsia. At the mental and emotional level the materia medica speaks of worry, especially for family, for one's children, and for business affairs. Also spoken of is miserable self-deprecation and two peculiar states: of not recognizing one's own children, and of "borrowing trouble." What does borrowing trouble mean? And how might the remedy picture's physical weaknesses and emotional worries be connected? Why does the Aceticum acidum individual worry so much about business affairs and the welfare of his family and children?

In other remedies where money worries are prominent the reason is clear:

- With Arsenicum album there is frugality due to a feeling that time is running out and the resources of members of the individual's circle of love must be safeguarded.
- A Bryonia person worries about the future due to his being materialistic but requiring support. Like the vine the remedy is made from, this individual seeks to climb to great heights but must cling to others who are depended upon for help in reaching specific goals.
- The Calcarea fluorica person is always running in place. This individual struggles to make financial headway.
- The Psorinum individual has a zealous internal accountant who constantly keeps track of incoming and outgoing resources.

The following case study will help shed light on the Aceticum acidum individual's worries.

Case Study
....
Shedding Light on Aceticum acidum

A client who reported needless but unceasing worry about his business perplexed me. He had already had or clearly did not need any of the remedies mentioned above, was self-deprecating, suffered from stubborn gastric problems, and seemed adept at causing himself uncalled-for mischief (borrowing trouble). I suspected Aceticum acidum but was troubled not to clearly understand his remedy condition. In the course of our consultation he offered something that seemed to shed light on the remedy's theme: My client's father, who had been adopted into a wealthy family, failed repeatedly to meet the family's expectations for responsible behavior. When the patriarch died the father inherited a fortune. But then, because my client's father remained irresponsible and was profligate in his spending, the family grew alarmed. Looking to rein him in, the executor for the family's estate stipulated a penurious stipend. For years thereafter and all through the town he was known as "the poor little rich man."

It occurred to me that my client's anguish evinced entanglement with his father's trauma. The Aceticum acidum remedy's working for my client indicated that I was right. Moreover, the remedy's effectiveness suggested its theme. A psoric quandary was at hand: Access to money to which one is entitled is denied. The theme boils down to *disenfranchisement*. Existential stress related to being disenfranchised is what underlies the pathology associated with Aceticum acidum.

The example of Aceticum acidum also reminds us that the homeopathic materia medica's expansion depends not just on provings (that convey what subjects in whom a remedy state has been inculcated report) but on practitioner observations as well. My client could show no worry for his children as he had none. Did the absence of this feature disqualify him for Aceticum acidum? No, because he never wanted to have children. He believed that parenthood necessarily entailed enacting cruelty upon one's children. My client's delusion that to be a father means being a brute upgraded my understanding of self-deprecation associated with Aceticum acidum.

Arsenicum album

With death inevitable, cling to what is of value

No margin for error	Aging and deterioration
Death obsession	Exhaustion
Anxious for those within circle of love	Heat within, cold without

We revisit a remedy discussed previously within the context of Fire and tubercular miasm. Taken to its logical conclusion, a sense that the world will not sustain my existence denotes expectation of death. Arsenic immediately follows phosphorus in the periodic table's group 15. In homeopathic microdosage this deadly chemical is deservedly famous for its ability to reverse intractable anxiety. Underlying all anxiety encountered in Arsenicum album patients is a preoccupation with and fear of death. Arsenicum individuals are fastidious, frugal, dependent on, and enmeshed with their family and caregivers. They can be obsessed with health, disease, or aging and decay. Tending to be perfectionists and tormented by the possibility of error, Arsenicum album individuals make excellent project coordinators and office managers who feel "I am the one who reliably gets it done."

Not surprisingly, Arsenicum album treats a variety of digestive complaints. It is almost a specific remedy for high-achieving, perfectionist schoolgirls suffering from anorexia nervosa. The fathers of such girls are often demanding, exacting high standards of excellence, a circumstance that illuminates the nature of challenge within the remedy and its radical disjunct: *I crave a state of perfection so as to stave off death, but when I achieve this state I perceive the stagnated nature of the perfected state, and this creates further terror of death.*

The following anorexia nervosa case exemplifies this theme.

Case Study
....
Arsenicum album for a Young Girl with Anorexia Nervosa

Thirteen-year-old Cecilia is a "perfect" girl, beloved by her friends, an excellent student, fine gymnast, fastidious in her appearance. She admits to having no symptoms whatsoever. Yet alarming weight loss and refusal to eat prompt her dismissal from the school gymnastics team, the only disappointment she acknowledges. Cecilia otherwise maintains that she has no symptoms or worries. In fact, she has no idea why she has been brought to my office.

Persistent questioning elicits the confession that on occasion she gets a stomachache. I ask how it feels. She tells me the sensation feels like an inward collapse of the stomach.

My prescription of Arsenicum album 200C will not surprise the experienced homeopath. Yet the girl's intransigence, her refusal to admit anxiety, fatigue, or perfectionism, merits discussion. A rubric, "sensation as if collapsing inward" is interpreted by me as a desire to retreat to the safety of the womb. Cecilia's subconscious agenda of reaching this safe haven via starvation is, of course, mad, a delusion encompassing the totality of her pathology. Refusal to eat, suggesting that *any* bite is more than she can chew, not to mention the weakness or unwillingness of her stomach to break down foodstuffs, implicates aggravation within the dimension of Taste.

Cecilia's Arsenicum album response was curative and retrospectively confirmed by both analysis and remedy prescription. She began to eat normally, but to the horror of her parents and siblings, Cecilia uncharacteristically also began to speak her mind, behave rebelliously, and generally bring upset to her family's emotional ecology. Several things became clear:

- Cecilia's main concern had been her family members' well-being (Arsenicum album and Taste's anxiety).
- Her prime obligation to protect family members (Arsenicum album's tight circle of love) required accepting the challenge of

maintaining a discipline of keeping her mouth shut (perversion of challenge within Taste and Arsenicum album's perfectionism).

• Although engineered to deflect her family from its troubles, Cecilia's pathological strategy imperils her own life (Arsenicum album's affinity with death).

These elements plus her teen age place the case squarely within the sense dimension of Taste.[2]

If anorexia nervosa is an extreme state of anxiety, many less dire conditions featuring anxiety will confront the busy homeopath. When prescribed appropriately, the remedy seldom fails to ameliorate an anxious condition and its excessive concern regarding death. Along with that, the digestive complaints, skin issues, chill (as in Reynaud's syndrome), and exhaustion will also improve.

Hair styling can be a homeopathic clue. For example, Natrum muriaticum women, because they hate to draw attention to themselves, are prone to low-maintenance and practical hairstyles. What I have noticed among Arsenicum album women is an affinity for the helmet-like, pageboy hairstyle that seems to cry out "I can get it done." As an in-service lecture I had the opportunity to explain Arsenicum album to some thirty members of a therapy practice. Describing the Arsenicum album personality as someone who would make an ideal office manager, I pointed to a woman standing in the back of the room who sported a pageboy haircut, saying she could look like that. Amazingly, I had in fact identified the office manager.

Calcarea carbonica

When will it all come together for me?

Analytical/cautious	Quickly out of breath
Overwhelmed	Sweaty/damp head
Easy weight gain	

Why is Calcarea carbonica, made from oyster shell, such an important remedy? The answer is its existential significance. At the moment we are born we are, each of us, a naked oyster, vulnerable and longing for a protective covering that went missing upon our emergence from the womb. The protective housing of an oyster's shell is composed of calcium and carbon, elemental building blocks of most of our body's structures. A revealing feature of the Calcarea carbonica remedy is its affinity for the fontanels of the skull that early on in an infant's development must conjoin so that the "roof" over the infant's head closes and protects the brain. Primal anxiety around this conjoining of the skull bones, a worry that unless the knitting together of the segments is complete the roof will leak and allow cold and damp, inspires the remedy's theme of "When will it all come together for me?" Susceptible to being overwhelmed by the high-stakes issue of his safety and security in the world, the Calcarea carbonica person is analytical, breaking problems into their constituent parts and asking metaphysical questions about life's purpose. Aware of the many steps that attend the securing of his safety, he makes lists as a coping mechanism. In a vicious cycle I call a radical disjunct, the coping mechanism not only fails to help but worsens matters for him. The numerous items on his list become his undoing as they generate even more reason to be overwhelmed.

In the worst periods the Calcarea carbonica individual has the sensation of flying apart at the seams, going crazy, or missing a single, overriding principle by means of which existence on earth can be explained. The Calcarea carbonica state's subtle defect that causes ready gain of weight, chill and susceptibility to cold, clamminess, shortness of breath, or excessive or insufficient sweat reflects the metabolic and generally binding significance of calcium.

Having personally experienced and been made ill by the extraordinary humidity in the part of China where I stayed (a nasty case of bronchitis), I will attest that damp is more than a metaphoric descriptor. Also known as a stationary obstruction in TCM, damp pertains to a fixed and localized pain, where the body and limbs feel heavy, often numb, with a tendency to edema.

Following a constitutional dose of Calcarea carbonica, an individual's metabolism gains efficiency. He is able to lose weight, gains stamina, generally feels warmer, and is less prone to becoming overwhelmed. As the affinity for dampness (external) and swelling (internal dampness) decreases, arthritic pain is ameliorated as well.

Camphora

Left out in the cold

Cold, chilled	Pain in the muscles and fasciae
Insensitive to input	Feels rejected
Raving	Antidoting

One of the most classically existential remedies, Camphora represents and treats total aloneness, a state of being "frozen out." This is an extreme expression of nonsustainability within the world. Prior experience of profound rejection from within the primary family is likely at cause, and also, perhaps, as we shall soon see, an earlier bout with a debilitating condition. At the physical level Camphora is an emergency remedy especially suited to ailments produced by violent causes. These can include overpowering infection, sudden chill, exposure to heat of the sun, trauma, the shock of a surgical procedure, or weakness following eruptions or discharges. It manifests with sudden and violent onset, extreme anxiety and restlessness, raging delirium, surging prostration, icy coldness, sopor (unusually deep sleep), and unconsciousness. Accompanying symptoms include cold sweat, nausea, vomiting, coffee grounds–like stools, cramps in the calves, and tetanic and epileptiform convulsions.

The muscles and fasciae will be found withered in someone needing this remedy (think of a snowman with twigs for arms). In parallel with its inherent sense of rejection by others, the remedy is famous as an antidoting substance. As if reenacting its "I am rejected" theme, Camphora rejects all other remedies.

Remarkably, Camphora has a very brief time frame, meaning that within a few days of its being prescribed, the patient does not instantly become a happy camper but a less dire picture emerges. Not uncommonly the change invokes a complementary remedy, Carbo vegetabilis, that as opposed to featuring emotional devastation presents primarily as prostration, a state of having to push through exhaustion to get anything done. A peeling away of the "onion skin" Camphora remedy layer so as to expose a Carbo vegetabilis layer suggests something else: The client likely earlier in life had undergone a debilitating condition. Never having been completely resolved, its characteristic prostration is now revisited, or the prior condition is retrospectively understood as having instigated susceptibility to the Camphora remedy state in the client.

Clematis recta

Just give me one thing I can hold on to

Anger at memory loss	Aversion to reading
Confusion/indifference	Neuralgia
Prostration	Glands, eyes, urethra
Peevish	Melancholy

An often-overlooked remedy, Clematis recta offers a meaningful subtext to psora's anxiety that *my existence is not sustainable.* With aging, memory becomes less and less reliable. It is fortunate that in Clematis recta there exists a remedy to address so poignant and universal a problem: the fear, anger, and actuality of memory loss. Memory loss can fuel or reflect Clematis recta's overriding issue of having nothing to grasp. The remedy state's melancholy and feeling of being unanchored are beautifully evoked by a John Prine song, "Angel from Montgomery."

> *Just give me one thing that I can hold on to,*
> *To believe in this living is just a hard way to go.*

The unanchored feeling of having nothing to hang on to manifests as melancholy, preoccupation with sad thoughts, despairing mood, indifference, silence and emptiness of thought, low spiritedness, peevishness without a cause, and, though desiring company, disinclination to meet even agreeable people.

Though Clematis recta is best known as a remedy for the urogenital system, skin ailments signaling not being okay in the world are prominent. These include itching over the whole body, a sticking sensation when touching skin, a gnawing sensation in the skin that scratching fails to ameliorate, skin redness, burning, and eruption of blisters that burst and form ulcers. Vesicles and pustules are seen to erupt, and watery secretions, scabs, and scales may manifest.

To suppose that a dose of Clematis recta will transform the client into an entirely happy camper is unreasonable. More reasonable to expect in addition to improved memory is amelioration of the physical symptoms, a departure from the sense of having nothing to hold on to, and emergence into a remedy state with a more clearly defined issue.

For example, Clematis recta's two principal complements are Mercurius vivus (or solubilis), a paranoia remedy (in the sense of being surrounded by enemies), and Silica (oversensitivity to impressions, orientation to small details, self-consciousness, and timorousness). To truly "graduate" from a remedy obligates the succeeding remedy to address remaining (or overlapping) symptoms. Depending on the individual's layering, not just Mercurius vivus or Silica but other remedy states can emerge.

Cobaltum metallicum
Existential guilt

My criminality is public knowledge
Personal insignificance
Self-reproach
Desire for mental work
Testicular pain and psychosexual dysfunction
Disordered gastrointestinal function
Respiratory issues

In March 2014, 2.7 million Chevy Cobalt cars were recalled, but not before they were tied to at least thirteen deaths. As noted earlier in this text, I would have advised General Motors that Cobalt was an unfortunate choice for a name. The word derives from the German *Kobold,* meaning "goblin." It was so named because in the eighteenth century, when it was discovered, the metal cobalt had no discernible use beyond its blue color and was deemed undesirable. Today, cobalt is a rare metal in demand in computer technology. The remedy's materia medica describes soreness of the throat and throat rawness attending repeated effort at expectoration. The Cobalt cough is short and hacking and can be accompanied by expectoration of bright red blood, issuing from the larynx.

The remedy made from cobalt heals individuals who feel as if they are guilty of a notorious crime and that their sinful act is public knowledge. This is exactly the fate that befell General Motors after news of the company's faulty ignition system could no longer be suppressed. Genuine criminals are unlikely to experience this remedy state. Assumption of responsibility or sense of guilt is precisely what "bad actors" typically lack. A strong example of the remedy Cobaltum metallicum would have been the subjects of famous Czech writer Franz Kafka. His writing opened a window into the anguish and guilt that the Cobaltum metallicum remedy state exemplifies.

Kafka's presence in the world was barely sustainable. As a boy he was frail and sensitive. His burly father was insensitive and hypercritical, and young Kafka experienced him as immensely threatening. Time and again in his fiction Kafka revisits the theme of a father, father-like, or authoritative figure emasculating and condemning a version of himself (the writer). In Kafka's first story, "The Judgment," a hypercritical father condemns his son to death, a directive with which the son dutifully complies by killing himself.[3]

Kafka's childhood trauma had a deranging effect, spurring dissociative mental activity and a sense of worthlessness and impotence. Within Traditional Chinese Medicine, worrisome mental activity disharmonizes the Spleen, disorders digestion (as in a sour stomach), or causes excessive production of phlegm (from which the writer suffered). In Kafka's case, phlegm production apparently rendered him susceptible to tuberculosis. On the positive side of the Cobaltum metallicum remedy state, it suggests remarkable resilience and persistence in the face of hardship, such as Franz Kafka, despite his heightened sensitivity, personified.

Falco peregrinus
I am shackled

Resistant to domesticity

Susceptible to captivity, lack of control in life

Detachment; cold anger; floating sensation

Sympathetic/clairvoyant

Scorned/undervalued

Wildness/childishness

Strong fingernails

Powerful eyesight

Cramping

Numbness/paralysis

Ravenous upon eating; nausea

Birds are the class of Aves, warm-blooded vertebrates whose chief characteristics are feathers; toothless, beaked jaws; the laying of hard-shelled eggs; a high metabolic rate; a four-chambered heart; and a strong yet lightweight skeleton. Challenged by the question, *Is my presence in the world sustainable?* their response is: "Not so much. Better to escape the earth and the proximity of its predators. I choose to evolve so as to attain the freedom of the sky."

In his insightful book *Birds: Seeking the Freedom of the Sky* Peter Fraser points out that the birds constitute "an evolutionary summit of the enormous reptilian branch of the tree of life that includes or included all the dinosaurs. . . . The birds have adapted not only to using the Realm of the Sky but they have made it their home and are completely comfortable in a place that was not originally theirs."[4]

Among the many interesting facts about birds that Fraser relates, accommodating to the sky has come at a cost and involved metabolic and structural design tradeoffs. For example, body weight has had to be minimized while large reserves of energy must be readily available.

So as to not impair their center of gravity while in flight, brain size has had to be kept relatively small. The birds thus rely less heavily on cognition-driven choice and more on instinctive behavior, while leaning on the support of one another in groups. We note that in remote locations where there is a dearth of predators birds can afford to evolve toward having bigger bodies and flightlessness.

The Falco peregrinus remedy, my lone remedy representative from the bird kingdom, was prepared from the blood and feather of a peregrine tiercel, a bird bred in captivity that had been trained to hunt in the traditional manner.[5] The peregrine falcon is the fastest-moving creature on earth and also a top-of-the-food-chain predator. Within mythology the falcon reflects supremacy and a wherewithal to transcend difficulties. For North American Indigenous peoples the falcon is a messenger conveying guidance from the spirit world. For the ancient Egyptians the falcon shepherded the sun's movement from morning to night. Falco peregrinus's freedom and power juxtaposed with its centuries-long history as a captured hunter within the practice of falconry render the remedy's affinity for extremely polarized tendencies understandable.

Affinity for Subjugation and Rage against Opposition

In keeping with the political nature of the sense dimension of Taste, Falco pereginus comes up for individuals who feel controlled and dominated by a parent, partner, lover, or offspring. The individual is likely to feel put down, humiliated, undervalued, and scorned. As if tethered to the falconer's arm, access to the wide sky comes with an iron-clad constraint, since the individual is forced to obey an overwhelmingly powerful force. This promotes a detached mindset, cold anger, numbness, and a sense of paralysis. By way of counterbalance the remedy state includes a sense of wildness, childish playfulness, concentrated focus, sympathy, clairvoyance, and strong fingernails. In keeping with the theme of psora, denied control of self-nurturance affects metabolism, causing ravenous hunger and nausea.

In my clinical experience I have seen Falco peregrinus help individuals break free from the emotional bondage of a longstanding obsessive and unfulfilling relationship.

Kali bichromicum

Excessively sustained

Stuckness in sinuses	Stuck in family
Stuckness in stomach	Thoughtless staring
Complacent	Poor concentration

Though this remedy is commonly invoked for acute conditions involving sinus congestion, it has a bigger picture. According to renowned author and homeopath Rajan Sankaran, needing the Potassium bichromate remedy indicates having been harmed by a family member and afterward, rather than experiencing anger, reacting with sadness and annoyance. The withholding aspect of the remedy picture reflects a theme associated with the remedy's chromium component. The Chromium remedy pertains to the maintenance of a nonthreatening facade so that public expression of negative feelings is constrained. Sankaran describes such people as unexpressive, taciturn, emotionally suppressed, avoidant of society, and generally hard. There is also an opposite sort of Kali bichromicum individual whom Sankaran describes as timid, bashful, apprehensive, anxious, and unconfident.[6]

Such individuals are also discouraged, averse to business, and sometimes unable to recognize their relatives. Both types of Kali bichromicum clients manifest stuckness, not only at the psychological level but also with regard to physical symptoms.

Case Study

Kali bichromicum
and a Curious Case of ADD

A version of the Kali bichromicum remedy state I have encountered involves imposition of an existential stress by a family member serving to induce the remedy's characteristic stuckness in the guise of an unusual attention deficit disorder (ADD). Let us call the thirteen-year-old child Ned. At the age of eleven Ned was diagnosed with eosinophilic esophagitis (EOE)—a stuckness condition involving white blood cell buildup in the esophagus, which his doctor controls with omeprazole.

Rather than being distractible, as the majority of such children are, Ned would become stuck on the topic or task garnering his attention and then would require strenuous efforts from his mother or father to redirect him to anything else. Though monomania or hyper-focus are typically at cause in such cases, neither describe this child. Ned's trancelike descent into nondistractibility displays instead the opposite of focused attention: indifference and complacency. Feeling zero compunction to leave the space in which he finds himself, Ned is content to occupy his current space indefinitely.

What might account for Ned's curious ADD? A backstory concerning Ned's mother's pregnancy holds a clue. Following several arduous pregnancies with his older siblings, Ned's mother had a curiously pleasant experience carrying Ned in her womb, during which time she was ravenously hungry, gained weight, and craved apple pie. She noted it was a rare interval when everything felt right in her life and she enjoyed a contentment bordering on the euphoric. In fact, she felt perfectly content and in need of nothing.

My conjecture, borne out by a successful prescription of Kali bichromicum (with improvement in his ADD), is that Ned became victimized by too much of a good thing. The inadvertent harm done to him by a family member involved an excess of nurturance in the womb. Deactivation of Ned's investment in his own sustenance resulted. This is not to suggest that every fulfilling, enjoyable pregnancy will produce a child needing Kali bichromicum. That would be ridiculous. Why it occurred in Ned's case, it is above my pay grade to understand, but the blueprint of Ned's life includes engaging with a state of utter contentment.

Ned's condition brings to mind a fictional character, the Russian novelist Ivan Goncharov's Ilya Ilyich Oblamov (from the novel Oblamov). A nobleman averse to society, Oblamov is so filled with indecision that he is unable to take any significant action. For large portions of the novel Oblamov fails to leave his room or bed.

Kali bromatum

Failure to meet God's standards

Melancholic and remorseful	Stammering
Bemoaning fate	Acne and boils
Hand-wringing/twitching	Sexual frustration
Dyspepsia	

When an individual has been brought up in a religious household or an environment espousing puritanical values, running afoul of its demanding norms can be dire. A judgment of being morally deficient and "on the outs" with God can result. This calls into question the basic right to sustenance. Here we have the Kali bromatum individual who, following sudden anger, fright, emotional disturbance, business loss, embarrassment, or guilt over sexual excess or sexual abuse, comes to feel singled out for God's punishment. The shame need not be expressed explicitly. Its presence is conveyed by hand-wringing and contorted speech, such as stammering. The presence of cystic acne (expressive of the psoric miasm) offers visible evidence of "unsuitability" before the eyes of God.

Kali bromatum is used to treat paranoid delusions, a feeling of helplessness, insecurity, a bad conscience, and aphasia and loss of memory. Physical symptoms also include numbness, impotence, dyspepsia, fidgeting, a stumbling gait, prostration, and seizures. The existential uplift this medicine provides is difficult to deny.

Lycopodium clavatum

Not yet ready

Compliant/controlling	Impotent/promiscuous
Insecure/distractible	Eating disorders
Horror of public speaking	

Millions of years ago in the carboniferous period of the late Paleozoic Era, the clavatums were tree-sized. With the advent of the taller and sturdier gymnosperm trees, these gigantic mosses must have decided that shrinking themselves to a height of some three inches served an evolutionary purpose. Consider this development as we discuss club moss, from which the Lycopodium clavatum remedy is derived.

Lycopodium embodies a theme of personal unreadiness rooted in a universally experienced happenstance: that each of us was once small and towered over by our much taller parents and older siblings. In normal development a sense of this height and power disparity falls away. When it does not, a sense of insignificance, incompetence, and unreadiness lingers. Due to a delusion that interaction with others always involves someone winning and someone losing, the Lycopodium person tends to feel powerless. Feelings of inadequacy are compensated for by controlling behavior or involvement in power-invoking activities such as the martial arts. Feeling out of control, the individual will balance a tendency to binge on carbohydrates or sugar with radical dieting. The Lycopodium clavatum man or woman may be a coward or a bully or some combination of both. A woman will often be a people pleaser.

Lycopodium clavatum can be relied on to shepherd insecure, distractible, and immature individuals on the path to maturity and confidence. Since a lone speaker confronts a multitude during public speaking, the situation is terrifying to the Lycopodium clavatum person. On the other hand, the lone individual who feels in control of a large audience will have a feeling of power because now this person is a winner.

Lycopodium clavatum people can also experience anxiety in open spaces (where their *I am insignificant* hot button is pushed) or in confined environments such as elevators, where a sense of being squeezed into a corner is strong. In keeping with Taste's challenge-anxiety axis, the Lycopodium clavatum individual, despite feeling intimidated or overmatched, is drawn to a challenge and either buckles under or fights back like a cornered rat. In keeping with psora, the remedy state disorders the gastrointestinal system, producing excessive gas and heartburn. It can also account for asthma and shortness of breath and compromise circulation, causing Reynaud's syndrome. It plays a role in a variety of reproductive complaints and, not surprisingly, in impotence and/or philandering.

Our familiarity with the typical gateway to the Lycopodium state sheds further light on the sense dimension of Taste. Lycopodium clavatum teaches us the equivalence of empowerment, the acquisition of a core competence, and emotional security. For example, a child about to be weaned from the breast must gain a core competence that is both frightening and empowering. In gaining awareness that hunger is a separate and not always met need, the child must grow adept in making the presence of hunger known. In addition, the child must master ingestion of solid food. If the transition is at all traumatic, a feeling lingers that *I am not quite there yet.* The appetite then greatly enlarges and the child becomes cranky and prone to colic.

A similar challenge awaits the child about to be toilet trained or who is learning to read. The child's awareness of limited competence fuels an excess of self-awareness that further subverts his ability to enter into the flow of a competence-based activity. Subconsciously comparing his reading skills with those of another child, he is now distracted from the book in his hands. Failing to absorb its contents, he spirals more deeply into self-consciousness.

One of my patients, an insecure and angry fourteen-year-old girl, offhandedly remarked that she first began having menstrual periods at the age of ten. In fact, early onset of menses is a Lycopodium clavatum keynote. For this girl, who at the age of ten was in no sense reproductively mature, menstrual precocity both signaled and predisposed her to an enduring Lycopodium clavatum remedy state.

Successful transition to a new core competence is empowering. An incomplete transition, on the other hand, compounds self-consciousness, producing a lingering immaturity that reinforces one's delusion of incapability, and incomplete development becomes a self-fulfilling prophecy. Lycopodium clavatum is a standby weapon not only against anxiety, but also against attention deficit disorder, reading disability, and a variety of appetite disorders.

Mezereum

Betwixt loyalties

> Anxious and mute
> "Vegetable Mercurius" (distilled essence)
> Stewing in my own juices
> Skin is crusty; lesions
> Head pain from suppressed anger
> Stomach pain from suppressed emotion

A universal and hard-to-sidestep life hazard is the imposition of being torn by opposing loyalties. Caught between conflicting loyalties, the individual needing Mezerium suffers an unendurable situation. For example, he may feel compelled to kowtow before an abusive relative from whom he stands to inherit. As if out of spite, this relative refuses to die! Stewing in his toxic juices, the would-be heir is stymied. The challenge is basically unmeetable.

In keeping with psora, Mezereum is primarily a medicine for skin disease accompanied by anxiety. The remedy's intense and varied skin presentation often includes suppuration and cracking and crusting of the lesions. The skin becomes dry and hot, with the flaking off of big patches. The Mezereum patient is usually serious-minded and often experiences an anguished or anxious epigastric sensation. Similar to a remedy called Phytolacca decandra, Mezereum is known as a "vegetable Mercurius vivus." This reflects a sharing with Mercurius of symptoms such as emotional closedness, bone pain, ear disorders, neuralgia, and skin diseases. Additional symptoms include a penetrating sensation in the occipital bones, acute ascending pains such as can draw a patient out of bed, right-sided occipital pain, discomforting ripping pain, throbbing in one spot above the nape, and stupefaction.

For someone suffering through chemotherapy (two loyalties: one to health, the other to the toxic medicines condemning him to literally stew in his own juices), low potencies of Mezerium should be considered.

Psorinum

What I have today will not suffice for tomorrow

Poverty consciousness	Itching/stinking
Accountant in the head	Chilly
Entrepreneurial	Eats like there is no tomorrow
Kvetching	

The psora miasm's nosode (made from the product of scabies) naturally enough is the remedy Psorinum, made from the scabies vesicle. Psorinum treats a variety of conditions, especially those of the skin. People needing Psorinum suffer from a specific kind of anxiety, often referred to as "poverty consciousness." They feel that they never have quite enough. The Yiddish language has a marvelous word, *bobkes,* that though denoting goat manure has colorfully come to mean "nothing," as in "I've got bobkes."

Rajan Sankaran describes the Psorinum individual as someone who is attempting to scale a mountain and has gotten stuck; with both options being too risky, he can neither ascend nor descend. Full of fear and despair due to having failed to properly assess the risks involved, rather than question the mountain itself, in tormenting fashion he doubts his own capability.[7]

As opposed to assessing his risks, the Psorinum individual endures the presence of a relentless internal accountant, a bookkeeper who obsesses about incoming remuneration—financial or otherwise—and depletion from the life account. The ledger is never balanced, hence there is endless complaining and a frightful anxiety about what the future may hold. Psorinum's materia medica includes voracious appetite, a symptom we can now decode: The individual needing Psorinum overeats out of a delusion of starving in the future. This person literally eats like there is no tomorrow.

Entrenched Expressions Embody Truths

When certain expressions become entrenched as idioms it is because they convey a universally familiar truth. For example, the craw is the crop or preliminary stomach of a fowl, where food is predigested. To say "this sticks in my craw" denotes when you can't swallow a food but also being loath to accept a wrongful circumstance. That such dissimilar symptoms link up within the human condition accounts for the idiom's entrenchment. Drosera rotundafolia is a remedy made from the carnivorous Venus flytrap, a plant whose nurturance requires digesting a protesting, buzzing insect. Since it addresses both the stuck-in-my-craw physical sensation and the trauma of betrayal by a family member or close associate, it is a homeopathic match for the idiom.

Going "blind with rage" is idiomatic but "deaf with rage" is not. The reason anger is associated with the sense of sight but not hearing is that sight and anger are entwined within our psyche, a connection hardwired within TCM theory. Likewise in Genesis Adam and Eve are evicted from the Garden of Eden because Eve first saw that the tree was good for food, was pleasant to the eyes, and would make one wise. She took the fruit and ate, also giving some to her husband to eat. Their consumption of the fruit drew an enraged reaction from God, who saw them hiding, seemingly out of sight behind a tree, and banished the couple from Paradise. The problem with sight is that it is panoramic. We always see more than we want. Envisioning a better world is one thing; bringing it about is another, since the imposition of change often angers those opposed to change or who do not hold the same vision.

In addition to options in acupuncture, homeopathy, and biomedicine, a range of therapeutic practices can help promote existential robustness within the sense dimension of Taste.

Taste Dimension Health Promotion Practices

- Chew and taste food thoroughly.
- Cook with care and artistry.
- Eat a nutritious, varied diet.
- Use local and seasonal foods.
- Nurture the mother of Taste, Touch: Maintain a regular spiritual practice.
- Exercise regularly.
- Experience hunger and satiety.
- Honor the feminine.
- Savor wisdom and knowledge.
- Identify, evaluate, and accept challenges.

3

Am I oriented in space and time?

Sycotic Miasm • Smell • Metal Phase •
Sadness • Lungs

What if I do not belong where I am placed? Who am I when deprived of my right to choose? Why do I lose myself in the excitement of the moment? Why is it so hard to stay in the moment? When grief is unbearable, shall I take up the hacksaw of sadness to escape the past's grip? These questions lie at the core of what I have termed the sense dimension of Smell. They also underlie our susceptibility to the sycotic (gonorrhea-related) miasm.

THE SYCOTIC MIASM AND THE
SENSE DIMENSION OF SMELL

The introduction of sycosis (from which Hahnemann's term "fig-wart disease" derives) is associated with the sexually transmitted disease gonorrhea. Gonorrhea's key feature is inflammation of the genitals that causes a constant or intermittent discharge. It infects both males and females and most often affects the urethra, rectum, or throat, though in females the cervix can also be affected.

When inherited as a miasm the sexual stimulation of the actual condition appears with the effect of generalizing the stimulation so that

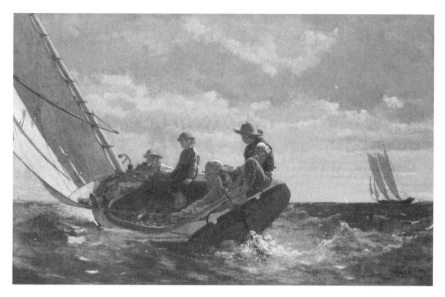

Breezing Up (A Fair Wind), painting by Winslow Homer

behaviors and emotions become infused with the wildness of sexual passion. It is as if one is stuck in the wild and addictive feeling of an orgasm, a place within which rational decision-making is difficult and where one's orientation in time is lost.

In the early 1960s America had a president, John F. Kennedy, who, given his sexual recklessness, outsized libido, and numerous debilitating conditions, which included Addison's disease and gonadal dysfunction, fits what is recognizably a Medorrhinum profile. Medorrhinum is a nosode made from the product of gonorrhea, a disease that, according to historian Robert Dallek, Kennedy likely contracted in his youth.[1] Kennnedy, Dallek reports, had "occasional burning when urinating, which was the result of a nonspecific urethritis dating from 1940 and a possible sexual encounter in college."[2] Some of the bacteria that cause this condition include E. coli, chlamydia, and gonorrhea.[3] Left untreated, the condition came to be described as "a mild, chronic, non-specific prostatitis" whose symptoms sulfa drugs suppressed. But as late as May 1955 Kennedy still had "prostatitis marked by pain when urinating and ejaculating, as well as urinary tract infections."[4]

An expression became popular within the sex, drugs, and rock 'n' roll culture of the late 1960s, reflective of sycosis's continuous genital discharge and disregard for possibilities latent within the present moment: "Hey man, go with the flow!" The recommendation to be laid back endorses openness to whatever comes your way. This invites burning the candle at both ends.

Though sycosis arises in a stealthy and subtle manner, with anemia and inflammation anywhere in the body, the miasm's eventual physical expression involves excess. Symptoms of excess include overgrowth of tissues causing warts, deposits in joints, and thickening of skin and nails, but also excitability counterbalanced by emotional suppression and a dearth of reactivity. The British homeopath and author Phyllis Speight offers the following as characteristic of sycosis:

- Headaches at vertex or frontal, worse after midnight, better from motion
- Snuffles in children; yellowing green catarrh from nose
- Musty or fishy taste in the mouth
- Face congested, blue; warty eruptions; facial hair falls out
- Fond of beer, rich foods, fat meats, and highly seasoned foods
- Abdominal pains better by hard pressure and bending double
- Tearing in joints, worse from rest and cold, damp weather
- Pain in small joints with infiltration and deposits[5]

The sycotic individual will be secretive, jealous, irritable, easily hurt, and rageful—characteristics we will relate to failure to resolve the core dilemma of centeredness versus disorientation in the sense dimension of Smell.

The Sense Dimension of Smell

Wuxing phase: Metal
Emotion: Grief/anguish
Organ: Lungs–Large Intestine–Skin (respiration)
Theme: Centeredness vs. disorientation

Smell is the chemical sense that enables us to detect signs and signals at a distance. This sense orients us to environmental conditions such as the smell of fire or oncoming rain. Scent markings tell of the presence of various animals. We locate plants by their fragrance, then imitate them with perfumes. Of all species, perhaps the most striking example of the orienting power of smell is the salmon, which depends on smell for guidance on the long journey back to its stream of origin to spawn.

By smell we identify and attract mates, communicate our emotional state, advertise the genotype of our immune system, signal illness, and bond with our kin. Each individual's smell signature is transiently influenced by foods consumed. A major component of flavor, smell contributes to the distinction between edible and inedible foods. As we are not conscious of each smell registered, many of our reactions are automatic as we are "led by the nose." The sense of smell's relevance to orientation and directionality comes from organic chemistry, where fragrance industry scientists have discovered that the nose assigns different odors to chemicals whose otherwise identical molecular structures are mirror images of one another. To the subtlest degree imaginable, the nose can tell right from left.

Smell occurs primarily through receptors in the nose, which sends signals processed by the brain. New genetic research suggests it is not odor receptors but the nervous system's wiring that actually determines how odors are defined. Powerfully linked with memory and emotion, smells have the ability to obliterate time. For example, whiffing the odor of a cigar re-creates childhood visits with a favorite uncle.

Smell orients imperceptibly as well. For example, chemoreceptors within sperm orient the sperm to the location of an egg. Less acute in humans than it is in mammals, the sense of smell may have been supplanted by increased acuity of vision and touch. With aging, humans lose some ability to smell; a significant majority of octogenarians have chronic dysfunction of smell. Sudden diminution of the sense of smell can forebode Alzheimer's disease. Moreover, the sense of smell declines markedly early on in the course of Alzheimer's dementia. Loss of sense of smell is also frequently mentioned in conjunction with the virus Covid, often persisting in long-haul Covid.

METAL PHASE AND
TRADITIONAL CHINESE MEDICINE

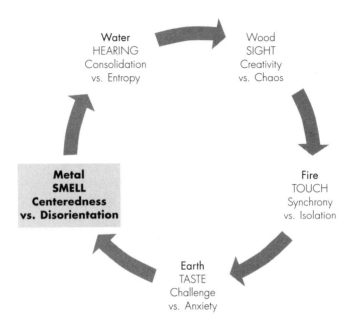

Water
HEARING
Consolidation
vs. Entropy

Wood
SIGHT
Creativity
vs. Chaos

**Metal
SMELL
Centeredness
vs. Disorientation**

Fire
TOUCH
Synchrony
vs. Isolation

Earth
TASTE
Challenge
vs. Anxiety

Within TCM's Wuxing the key emotion is sadness and the pertaining (solid) organ is the Lungs. This is understandable. When we are in grief, the chest that houses our lungs can become wracked with sobs. Entrenched grief, as we learned from the Inborn Toolkit, is reluctance to use the hacksaw of grief. It is also sycotic in that it expresses stuckness in time, inability to cut oneself free from the past.

Grief as the Emotion of Metal

One might think that depression arising from the deprivation of sunlight, namely seasonal affective disorder (SAD), is rooted in the sense dimension of Sight. I interpret SAD as expressing disorientation relating to Smell. The shortening of daylight hours in wintertime causes many of us to become blue, but the distress of the SAD individual can be overwhelming. Listless and depressed, he droops, much like a plant that fails to orient itself adequately to the sun.

Sunlight and water are key components of a respiration process known as photosynthesis, by which plants manufacture their own nutrients. It is fair to say that plants deprived of sunlight fear imminent starvation. Light-starved SAD individuals suffer the unbalancing of their master gland of homeostasis, the hypothalamus. As a result, regulation of numerous vital functions becomes problematic.

Biology and the Body's Emotional Climate

The hypothalamus's main function, to maintain our body's status quo, serves to ground our physical existence in the present moment. The hypothalamus creates and sustains set points for our blood pressure and skin temperature. It determines the threshold level of toxicity that our blood can carry, or that brain tissue can tolerate before detoxification by expulsive vomiting is prompted. Because the limbic and olfactory systems project to the hypothalamus, the gland plays a major role in regulating hunger and sexual desire. In regulating our circadian rhythms and synchronizing them with daylight and darkness, the hypothalamus also sets our sleep patterns.

We can rebalance the hypothalamus and overcome SAD by inhaling additional sunlight through the pores. By combining maximal outdoor activity with periodic indoor exposure to full-spectrum lighting similar to sunlight, we help our body recover its physical bearings. Inhalation of sunlight orients our body to the demands of the present moment.

Emotional Drooping

A homeopathic remedy, Sol, which is actually made from potentiated sunlight, belongs to a group of remedies (known as the Imponderables) made from energies such as X-rays and spectrum colors. Sol may be useful in dealing with disorientation resulting from both an excess of sunlight, as in heatstroke, and a deficiency, as in "sundowning" behavior observed among Alzheimer's disease individuals.

THE LUNGS AND
LARGE INTESTINE WITHIN TCM

The Lungs in TCM are conceived of as the ruler of the chi, which they help form and then distribute downward throughout the body. The Lungs govern respiration, bringing in pure chi and expelling impure chi. The Lungs receive nutritive fluids from the Spleen, and Lung chi moves and balances these fluids.

As the ruler of the body's exterior, the Lungs contribute not only to the condition of the skin but also to the defensive energy that protects the body from disease. Thus, in biomedical terms, the lungs provide immune system functions. The Lungs and their paired organ, the Large Intestine, belong to the phase of Metal, which is associated with autumn and with crying and grief (and here, the sense dimension of Smell).

The Lungs are said to house the *po,* or corporeal soul. In TCM the po is the equivalent of our bodily animal spirit. Thus the animating presence lives and dies with the body and is sustained with us through breathing. All breathing creatures have a corporeal soul, a mark of brotherhood among animal life forms. The signs and symptoms of Lung disorders in TCM include acute and chronic respiratory disorders, inflammation of the nose or throat, coughing, excessive phlegm, loss of voice, spontaneous sweating, allergies to airborne substances, and dry skin.

Disorders of the colon, such as constipation and irritable bowel syndrome, may be included because of the energetic link between Lungs and Large Intestine. Histologically the colon is a cylinder of skin. Ménière's disease, discussed within the context of the sense dimension of Hearing, includes a disorientation symptom, namely vertigo, that not surprisingly also reflects the pathology of the Lungs: Phlegm and dampness obstruct the Middle Burner (one of the six yang organs in the body), a metaphysical construct within TCM indicating the heart of the digestive system. The comparison is with a woodburning stove that heats a house: Digestion is the stove and food is the fuel. Within TCM the chi of respiration, also known as the cleansing yang chi, rises to the eyes, ears, nose, and mouth. To support the chi of respiration and clarity of the senses, Middle Burner suppression of phlegm must be stopped.

Respiration and Time

Respiration orients us to the past and the future. We take our first breath at birth, an inhalation of air and of the future before us. In death, a conclusive exhalation releases us from connection to past experience. In between birth and death, at an average of sixteen times a minute, we repeat this same activity that involves embrace of the future and release from the past. A qigong master believes that by mastering inward breath, allowing it to fully extend downward into the "cinnabar field" below the navel and within the abdomen (which the Chinese refer to as the *tan tien*), a kind of immortality or very long life is achieved, with all pathology postponed to the very end.

This does not mean someone cannot die, but rather that, having achieved mastery over all possibilities, the individual no longer worries about the future. The qigong master knows that mastering the extended, exhaled breath bodes freedom from attachment to the fleeting past and unencumbered participation in the life energy sparkling amid the emptiness of the universe. Ordinary language reflects an inherent linkage of inhalation and freedom within the context of independence. Thus the word "inspiration" denotes both the inhaled breath and receptiveness to astonishing ideas.

To follow the Tao means to seek mastery of both the inward and outward breath and therefore of the present, the future, and the past. It was often said in ancient times that to achieve the Tao matters less than setting out in the general direction of the Tao. This option and its attendant health benefits lie completely within the reach of ordinary people, not only qigong masters.

In the course of animal evolution, physiologic respiration moved from exterior surfaces to inside the body. Single-celled creatures exchange gases through cell wall surfaces; frogs conduct respiration through their moist skins. As an animal's size increases, the surface area of the skin becomes insufficient to support the greater requirements of gas exchange. The lungs in an adult human provide about seventy square meters of total surface area. Meeting these higher demands on physiologic respiration has drawn the location of breathing inward to the body's center.

There is also a connection between our psychological sense of centeredness and the locus of breathing. In panic attacks, breathing becomes rapid and shallow. This pattern of breathing may itself induce panic and the loss of grounding. Panic's decentering, in which the reptilian brain wrestles rational control away from otherwise in-charge, executive function, can be countered by focus on deep abdominal breathing.

CENTEREDNESS AND ORIENTATION

To be centered or oriented means to be aware of the self in present surroundings. This aspect of centeredness or orientation may be spatial, environmental, cultural, social, or spiritual. There is also a temporal aspect to orientation, an awareness of the present moment tempered by relevant history and future possibilities.

Orientation takes a decidedly interior turn with respect to breathing. With every breath we define our center by the depth of our relationship with the plenum of air, to which all other beings are simultaneously attached. The presence and penetration of the aromatic air orients us not only to all it conveys, but to our own central core. In a very real sense each inhalation draws forth the future. Each exhalation expels the past. Thus, mastery of breathing orients us in the present with respect to past and future. No wonder so many meditative practices emphasize attending to the breath, and that breath and spirit share the same linguistic root in so many languages. Breathing constitutes the foundation of centeredness.

Disorientation

This is the opposing pole to centeredness on this axis. Our compass may become skewed or utterly lost, leaving us unable to locate or balance self-interest and communal interest. We may fall into temporal distortions, grieving and unable to part with a preferred past, or frozen in terror by a traumatic event from years long past. Lacking resolution and inspiration, we limp through life like one wounded. This ingrained disorientation then manifests through symptoms of chronic illness.

Dementia

Alzheimer's disease, which may have genetic causes or be rooted in problems with amyloid beta protein and tau in the brain, is the most common cause of senility. The disease begins with difficulty learning or remembering recent events. Major depression can also cause senility, as can brain disorders. These disorders may be triggered by trauma, illness, or infection. A variety of conditions, such as Parkinson's disease, Pick's disease, Creutzfeldt-Jakob disease, vascular dementia, Huntington's disease, strokes, Down syndrome, head trauma, dementia with Lewy bodies, and AIDS can also cause senility. Senility associated with these conditions is generally irreversible.

Other conditions or illnesses that can cause senility include hypothyroidism, depressive pseudodementia, tumors, and normal pressure hydrocephalus. Deficiencies in vitamins B1, B12, and A as well as abuse of drugs and alcohol also cause an increased risk of developing senility. Similarly, individuals who inhale paint or other substances in order to get high may develop senility. Overmedication or dehydration may also cause a person to exhibit signs of senility and lead to a false diagnosis of Alzheimer's disease. Senile dementia is attributable to end-stage syphilis, the syphilitic diathesis within homeopathy, and environmental toxicity. Benzodiazepines (drugs that include anxiety medications and sleeping pills) and anticholinergics (a group encompassing medications for allergies and colds, depression, high blood pressure, and incontinence) are also associated with increased risk of dementia.

It may also result from the abominations of animal husbandry. The following section is from *Interpreting Chronic Illness:*

Prions, or "proteinaceous infectious particles," are peculiar and unique disease-causing proteins found by the neurologist Stanley B. Prusiner in the early 1980s, which he called "PrP," for prion protein. For reasons and by means as yet unknown, prions are able to invert their structure, replicate, and change their shape, converting normal protein molecules into dangerous ones. Known prion diseases, all fatal, are also called spongiform encephalopathies because the proliferation of prions leaves gaping holes in the brain tissue of mammals. The most common form, found in sheep and goats, is called "scrapie," a term arising from the animals' need to scrape off their wool or hair because of an intense symptomatic itch. Bovine spongiform encephalopathy—Mad Cow Disease—was identified in cows in Great Britain in 1986; the source of the disease was found to be a food supplement fed to the cows made from ground carcasses of cattle and sheep that may have been infected with a brain-wasting disease.[6]

When we foist a carnivorous and cannibalistic diet on vegetarian cattle, our species shows disdain for the great circle of life encompassing cattle and all other animals. Disdain for our humble position within nature's kingdom denotes spiritual loss of reference. My conjecture is that consuming meat from abominably treated cattle ushers us into madness: Alzheimer's disease with its characteristic loss of reference.

The Sycotic Miasm's Existential Themes

- Lost in time
- Disorientation of identity
- Disoriented in space
- Led by the nose
- Grief/shame/guilt
- Secretiveness
- Addictiveness

TREATMENTS AND EXPECTATIONS

Remedies manifesting subcategories of *Am I oriented in space and time?*

Acacia seyal	Natrum muriaticum
Alumina	Natrum sulphuricum
Borax	Nux moschata
Cimicifuga racemosa	Sabina
Hydrastis canadensis	Samarium
Lachesis muta	Senega
Lilium tigrinum	Sepia
Lithium carbonicum	Thuja occidentalis
Medorrhinum	Viscum album

Acacia seyal

Make me a coffin

Stuck in a transition state

Foggy, empty mind

Fatigue, lethargy

Boredom

Sensitive nose, nose as soul exit point

Baby unwilling to be born

Sinus congestion

Cannot choose between life and death

Afterlife concern

When a dying client is suffering during transition to the next world, two homeopathic remedies can be employed to facilitate the passage. (Note: this does not mean euthanizing.) The remedies are high potencies of Arsenicum album and Phosphorus. Acacia seyal now offers a third option.

The remedy treats a sycotic disorientation expressed by the feeling *I am somewhere between birth and death, but it's not clear where.* Related existential questions pertain to this medicine made from a tall African desert tree with a yellow-orange trunk: *Am I alive or am I dead? Do I even want to live? If I am about to die, what comes next? Is there an afterlife or a resurrection?* Entry to this state could occur subsequent to severe trauma or a near death experience.

Acacia seyal's extra-tough xylem was used by early Egyptians to fashion coffins. According to Michal Yakir, who proved the remedy made from this botanical in 2014, it is widely assumed that its wood was used to build the Ark of the Covenant. Not surprisingly, images and thoughts of coffins were prominent during its proving. Drawing on Arthur Cronquist's botanical classification approach, a pre-genetic, phenotype system that preceded the introduction of the APG (Angiosperm Phylogeny Group) system of taxonomy, Dr. Yakir interprets Acacia seyal as embodying "existential insecurity, isolation, paralysis, and dread of work." This reflects an oral stage of development wherein strong bonding with a mother has not occurred.[7]

Accordingly, the remedy state presents with fatigue, lethargy, boredom, and mental vacuity. The sense of not wanting to be born recommends its appropriateness for delivery problems in the birth canal. Further indicating its placement in the sense dimension of Smell, we find congestive nose and sinus symptoms, delusion of odd smells like the smell of a coffin, and imagery and thoughts about the soul's leaving the body through the nose.

From the standpoint of "not being entirely here," we can compare Acacia seyal with Lac maternum, a remedy made from the milk of nine different mothers. Due to not having ever been nursed, individuals needing Lac maternum do not fully incarnate, exhibit poor concentration and a lack of joy, and have trouble forming good relationships. The differentiation with Acacia seyal would be that these individuals are in no way concerned with death or afterlife.

Noting that Acacia seyal belongs to the Fabaceae family, Yakir, in collaboration with Ronan Levy and Koby Nehushtan, describes its subdivision the Fabales (Leguminales) as:

> [Living] in symbiosis with root fungi that serve as nitrogen fixers, reflecting the theme of "nurture by the Other." Legumes are high in protein and therefore highly nutritious, which again represents the Order's theme and tendency towards digestive symptoms. The pod structure is likewise reminiscent of home and family ties.[8]

Yakir describes the Fabales order in terms of:

> *Existential insecurity; the other person perceived as threatening, dangerous or oppressive; dominance vs submission; expression of aggression.* The combination of existential insecurity with the escalating presence of the masculine creates a sense of threat that may turn into full-blown paranoia. There is a strong sense of being oppressed and a dynamic of dominance and submission that elicits a hostile reaction. In the physical realm there will be congestion, hardening and atherosclerosis.[9]

The Fabaceae family and Fabales include two remedies whose representation of existential insecurity and personality weakness indicates their use in treating paralytic disease. The first is Cicer arietinum, effective for nervous system weakness and multiple sclerosis but also lithiasis, a condition predisposing liver damage, jaundice, and stony sediments in the body. The second is Lathyrus sativa, whose representation of a lack of trust, desire to escape, and sense of persecution enables the remedy to treat conditions such as polio (also as a polio preventive), multiple sclerosis, muscular dystrophy, and Parkinson's disease.

Alumina

Compromise of the will

Confusion/dementia	Don't like my choices
Overwhelmed	Cannot be hurried
Loss of reference	Violent impulse
Numbness of extremities	

An Alumina remedy state can result from exposure to aluminum but can also be transmitted by means of eating contaminated meat. It was long thought that despite sharing dementia as a common symptom, Alzheimer's disease and spongiform or brain-wasting diseases, notorious for their transmittal by consumption of contaminated meat, had nothing in common. That has changed. A brain-wasting disease, Creutzfeldt-Jacob disease (CJD), can be passed along genetically as well. Until recently rarely seen among Western people, CJD primarily afflicts the elderly. In England in the 1990s there arose a frightening departure, new variant Creutzfeldt-Jacob disease (nvCJD), whose high incidence among the general population shocked everyone. Creutzfeldt-Jacob disease is now suspected to be both seriously underdiagnosed as a cause of death as well as often misdiagnosed as Alzheimer's disease.

When writing *Interpreting Chronic Illness* I classified Alumina as pertaining to the sense dimension of Smell. It did not surprise me afterward, to learn that a predictive feature of Alzheimer's disease is early diminution of the sense of smell. To be "oriented" literally means to be drawn to the East (if one resides in the Western world). The tendency of Alzheimer's patients to wander as the sun goes down, a behavior known as sundowning, is in concert with the orientation loss.

The Alumina state can also develop as a response to stressful life events. Individuals so affected manifest a powerful confusion, a feeling akin to having two heads. This is promoted from events having led them to compromise their will and suffer loss of independence. Evolution of the mindset invites neuropathology as well. Alumina, for example, has proved beneficial for an elderly woman in my care suffering from multiple sclerosis. As a young woman her marriage to a man she did not particularly care for had been engineered via a cabal involving the man himself and the unwilling bride's older sister.

The general symptoms of Alumina include inability to think connectedly, anxiety and peevishness, weakness of memory, poor sense of self, pessimism, alternating paroxysms of laughing and weeping, fear of losing track of thoughts and reason, sudden impulses to violence, and severe constipation.

Alumina and the Will

Though we call ourselves human beings, the lesson of Alumina seems to be that it would be more accurate to think of ourselves as "human doings." Conflating *what we will to do* with *who we are* is Arthur Schopenhauer, a pessimistic philosopher who places the will center stage, responsible for the tragedy of life. Schopenhauer proposes that it is the will's nature to seek satisfaction via the pursuit of goals. Yet despite its purposive force, the attainment of a goal set by the will never completely satisfies.

Symbolically and otherwise, it is with our hands that our will is implemented in the world. Numbness and tingling of the hands in the Alumina picture thus reflects or further promotes the Alumina individual's existential plight: Choices that have been offered are unsatisfactory. This individual has been forced to make an undesirable choice. Aversion to being hurried amounts to the same thing. Despite being unready to act, the individual is compelled to do so. One of my clients had been brought up to believe that emotions must be mastered by the will. An Alumina mindset in the form of her feeling constantly thwarted—opposed in her choices—ensued. The chronic constipation she suffered from also reflects Alumina's insistent plaint: "I [meaning the stool] won't be rushed!"

Borax

Don't put me down!

> Worse with downward motion
>
> Flinching from slight noises; waking from sleep, horrified and crying
>
> Aphthae; transparent and thick mucus discharges
>
> Worse before stool or micturition; better afterward
>
> Ailments of breastfeeding mothers and breastfed babies
>
> Worse lying on right side

Might an infant or toddler have an existential issue? The remedy Borax teaches us that yes, this is indeed possible. Because physical connection with the mother is of paramount importance to an infant, insecurity in regard to the reliability of being held can be traumatic for this small being. Through no fault of the parent the issue of insecurity can arise if, for example, a newborn has to spend time in an intensive care unit, or when hospitalization for treatment of a congenital defect or premature birth has deprived the infant of sufficient opportunities to be held. Borax teaches us that being "put down" in the crib reenacts the drama of physical abandonment. The association of being placed down with trauma reverberates in language with the idiomatic meaning of "a put-down," or severe criticism.

The Borax individual, usually an infant or toddler, is vertically disoriented in space. Made worse from falling forward (put down) but then also confused when raised up is a problem of vertical displacement. The disorientation is also sycotic since the Borax state reflects both attachment to the past, a traumatic experience of physical abandonment, and the manifestation of the remedy state's other primary symptom, copious discharges of transparent thick mucus. The materia medica notes also that a mother being in synchrony (and sympathy) with her newborn can benefit from a dose of Borax if she is experiencing difficulty with breastfeeding.

Cimicifuga racemosa

The imprisoning bond of motherhood

> Rheumatism, especially of the back and neck
>
> Loquacity
>
> Utero-ovarian dysfunction
>
> Feeling of being encaged by wires
>
> Aggravation from touch
>
> Hysteria (delusion of being enveloped by a black cloud)

Fortunately it does not happen in every instance, but the onset of awareness of what pregnancy entails is frightening: "I love my new-born, but oh my God! I am now tethered to this human being for the rest of my life!" Existential disorientation such as this defeats logical argument. The interplay of excitement and dismay underlies many instances of what is clinically called postpartum depression. Made from black cohosh, Cimicifuga racemosa is mainly a women's remedy. Its keynotes include loquacity, changeability, gloominess, muscle and nerve pain, uterine and ovarian dysfunction, an imprisoning sense of the chest being encaged by wires, and, in particular, a feeling of being engulfed by a black cloud. The remedy's power to dispel postpartum depression is a great gift.

Hydrastis canadensis

Furious at my declining memory

> Cannot remember what was read
>
> Mucosal inflammation
>
> Thick discharges
>
> Precancerous/marasmus (loss of adipose tissue from malnutrition)
>
> Malicious/nervous
>
> Depressed/sure of death

Imagine how you would feel if you suddenly could not remember what you had read. With aging, we are all condemned to varying degrees to experience memory deterioration. The Hydrastis canadensis mindset reflects or promotes the rage that can engulf us when faced with this existential problem. This remedy derived from goldenseal, also known as orangeroot or yellow puccoon, is made from the tincture of the fresh root. Its mental symptoms include forgetfulness, inability to remember what is being read or talked about, irritability, spitefulness, gloominess, taciturnity, moaning and crying out from pain, depression, and certainty of approaching death and longing for its arrival.

The head can feel as if intoxicated. There is dullness of the head, a heavy frontal headache over the eyes from catarrh, also causing a sharp cutting pain in the temples and over the eyes. Symptoms involve the eyes: profuse secretion of tears with smarting and burning of eyes and lids, blepharitis marginalis (itching and burning inflammatory condition of the eyes), thick mucus discharge, and dark greenish-yellow conjunctiva. As Hydrastis canadensis is a famous remedy for thick mucus congestion, it is not surprising that the ears are also involved, with otorrhea and a roaring, industrial type of sound in the ears. The ears can hurt, with pain extending to the forehead and over the eye. The remedy is useful in treating lumbago, emaciation, and prostration.

Hydastis canadensis is useful for ailments involving the Liver (in TCM associated with anger) but also with cancer and a cancerous state, especially before ulceration when pain is the principal symptom. Though a remedy we could just as easily catalog within the sense dimension of Sight and the cancer miasm, we place Hydrastis canadensis with Smell due to its value in dispelling mucosal inflammation and the disorienting effect of memory loss.

Lachesis muta

Civilization and its discontents

Thwarted primal instincts

Jealousy and suspicion

Alcoholism

Intensity, loquacity, clairvoyance

Manipulativeness

Heart ailments

Asthma

Sigmund Freud's book *Civilization and Its Discontents* presents the case that like other creatures on the earth, human beings are motivated by primal directives. These include desire for food, reproductively promising mates, and elevated status. Yet the drive to satisfy our desires is at odds with a social need to subjugate passions so that we do not commit murder, rape, theft, and so forth. Condemned to suppress their normal desires, human beings suffer existentially from the effort. As a result we must all struggle to subdue the inborn intensity of sexual possessiveness and envy. I would argue that Freud's gloomy philosophy fits not all human beings, only those in need of snake remedies such as Lachesis muta.

The materia medica of Lachesis muta, made from the venom of the Brazilian bushmaster snake, reflects how squashing of the instincts entails suffering of numerous ailments. Conflict erupting between the head that houses the ego, from which a suppressive agenda issues, and the body's trunk, wherein primal urges roil, creates sensitivity and inflammation in the battle zone located in between, namely, the neck and throat. Thus the Lachesis muta individual cannot bear to wear anything tight around the neck (elicits the subconscious image of a strangulating snake wrapped around the throat) and may have swollen neck lymph glands, difficulty swallowing, and a tendency to asthma and sore throat. In this pressure cooker, chest hypertension may erupt with attendant anxiety and the Lachesis muta person will self-sedate with intoxicants.

Though Lachesis muta also pertains to other miasms, I place it within sycosis by virtue of its prominence as a remedy for both asthma and skin eruptions (purple and bluish boils and carbuncles) and the fact that a gateway to the remedy state is grief; and a hysteria that manifests and is disorienting to the sense of time.

Lachesis muta is a remedy for individuals whose intensity lends itself to clairvoyance and attunement to the inner demands of primal desire. Thwarted by social pressure, these raw impulses are converted or sublimated into more generally acceptable behaviors, such as articulateness, singing, and loquacity.

Lilium tigrinum

Can my soul be saved?

Am I depraved?	Tearing of hair/cursing
Weeping made worse from consolation	Miscarriage
Moral despair regarding sinfulness	Multitasks

Society has long demanded that women be more pure-minded than men. This reflects the greater consequences women suffer when violation of spiritual norms produces inconvenient pregnancies. Hence Lilium tigrinum is prescribed more often for women than for men. The classical expression of its core theme, "tormented about her salvation," belies a confusion of identity. It typically reflects religious conflict concerning sexual thoughts, grief over a miscarriage, or some other unbearable, ethically charged grief. Fearing she is depraved, she rejects consolation. She is profoundly depressed, with a constant inclination to weep. In her anxiety she expects the onset of some organic and incurable disease. Caught in her intractable moral quandary, she curses, strikes out, and uses obscene language. Though her behavior is aimless, it is also hurried as she seeks relief in being occupied.

Awakening of the sexual instinct, especially among girls brought up in a religiously conservative or fundamentalist culture, will promote susceptibility to the remedy state. Though in the past Lilium tigrinum women undoubtedly pulled out their scalp hair, nowadays we are more likely to see the remedy's expression within an OCD presentation, such as pulling out of the eyelashes (trichotillomania). Bodily hair symbolically denotes untamed sexuality, for which reason someone in the Lilium tigrinum state plucks and pulls at it. On the flip side of untamed sexuality, the radical disjunct of hair removal, as in the trend of shaving body hair, reflects a hedonistic turn toward loosened sexuality or tactility.

Significant feelings include that of having a load on her chest and a cold feeling about the heart. In a crowded or warm room she will feel as though suffocating. Angina pectoris with pain in the right arm can appear in the Lilium state. Menses appear early and are scanty, dark, clotted, and offensive. The flow occurs only when she is in motion. There is a bearing-down sensation with urgent desire for stool, as though all organs want to escape. She may experience pain in the ovaries and down the thighs, with acrid, brown leukorrhea smarting in the labia. She may have a bloated feeling in the uterine region.

As opposed to an occasional concern, the issue of salvation has long been central to the lives of religious devotees. According to Jamie Kreiner in his book *The Wandering Mind: What Medieval Monks Tell Us about Distraction,* monks of late antiquity and during the years 300 to 900 CE struggled mightily against diversion while seeking to maintain chastity and a connection between their minds and God's.[10]

As Jennifer Szalai in her review of the book put it: "Swap out 'eternal life and death' for the bland mantras of 'productivity' and you'll get a sense of how the stakes for monks were quite different from ours."[11]

Tortured vacillation between aimless thought and frenzied prayer sounds like Lilium tigrinum. It also raises an existential issue pertaining to what is supposedly a scourge within modern education: attention deficit disorder (ADD). Casey Cep in her commentary on the book says: "Perhaps that is why so many of us have half-done tasks on our to-do lists and half-read books on our bedside tables, scroll through Instagram while simultaneously watching Netflix, and swiping between apps and tabs endlessly. . . . One uncomfortable explanation for why so many aspects of modern life corrode our attention is that *they do not merit it*" (italics mine). The real contribution of *The Wandering Mind,* she suggests, is that it takes us beyond the question of why the mind wanders "to the more difficult and more beautiful question of where it should rest."[12] I find myself wondering, would it be better if our children more frequently required Lilium tigrinum than "seriously distracted" remedies such as Fluoricum acidum and Cannabis indica?

Lithium carbonicum

What shall I do with my life?

Feeling useless

Weakness of the will

Frequent shifting of work and locale

Weeping from lonely condition

Having an undependable father

Ailments of the eyes, heart, small joints, and urinary organs

Rheumatism

Whole body sore and heavy

A subset of the sycotic question *Am I oriented in space and time?* is the existential question *What shall I do with my life?* The query is not unfamiliar. Each of us has at one time or another asked the question. It often crops up during college or in our early twenties when we are compelled to commit to one kind of work or another. But if it remains in place and torments us beyond situational choice, something is amiss. Unappealing or limited options in the workplace environment don't account for the distress. An issue embedded in Lithium carbonicum does. The remedy teaches that what is to blame is an undependable father, a male parent whose changeable nature has made him unreliable.

Lithium carbonate, from which the remedy Lithium carbonicum derives, is a synthesis of lithium salts with soda or potash. Incorporation of lithium carbonate in lithium-ion batteries enhances their power and application. The function of a battery is to contain and consolidate power. As homeopathy is the realm where the metaphorical is literal, the carbonate presence is understood to represent masculine energy as it pertains to structure and willpower. When carbonicum appears within the name of a homeopathic remedy, this expresses a need for structure, stability, and a bolstering of identity. The father of someone in need of Lithium carb is the insubstantial "positive pole" of a battery. As such, he is at fault for poor consolidation of the battery's power and the lack of willpower and wherewithal of his child. Commitment to a career pathway requiring willpower and wherewithal is precisely what the Lithium carbonicum individual lacks.*

The Lithium carbonicum person feels useless, is prone to frequent change of occupation, weeps from loneliness, and feels she does not know what to do with her life. In the background would be a father who was seldom home, or when at home was a vacillating and unreliable family presence. Her physical symptoms are likely to include eye problems, heart issues, urinary ailments, muscle knots, rheumatism, and feelings of tension and heaviness in the body.

Upon graduating from the Lithium carbonicum remedy state, the individual is likely to go into the remedy's complement, Lycopodium clavatum. If so, her sense of uselessness and lack of wherewithal will be downgraded to a state where she has gained a sense of what needs to be done but is insecure and unready to take the next step.

Medorrhinum

Sex, drugs, and rock 'n' roll

Reckless

Go with the flow

Loses track of conversation

Either all in or all out; rarely neutral

Foul odors

Heart ailments

Stuck in the orgasm (passionate excitement that overrules rational
thought)

---

*A remedy not discussed in this book, Zincum metallicum, treats a closely related problem. Zinc, like lithium, is a metal critical to the strengthening of alloys. It also functions to enhance the power of batteries. The individual in need of Zincum metallicum is a complainer, is prone to sudden loss of brain power, and is thrown for a loop by the most minor inconvenience. Most tellingly, the Zincum metallicum individual has or has had a remote relationship with their father.

Medorrhinum, the nosode derived from the gonorrhea virus, encapsulates what was said earlier about the sycosis miasm, in particular the reckless-ness, addictiveness, passion for what one cares about, and sensation akin to being stuck in an orgasm. Think of the early days of recreational drugs and sexual liberation. Pleasant as an orgasm is, it provides less than an ideal vantage point for rational thinking or centeredness with regard to time. Constantine Hering's list of symptoms makes this clear:

- Great weakness of memory. Dullness of memory and desire to pro-crastinate, because business seemed so long lasting, or as if it never could be accomplished.
- Entirely forgot what had been read, even previous line.
- Forgetfulness of names, later of words and initial letters.
- Cannot remember names: has to ask name of a most intimate friend; forgets own.
- Cannot spell correctly; wonders how the word "how" is spelled. Reads a letter and thinks the words look queer and are spelled wrong.
- Time moves too slowly.
- Dazed feeling; a far-off sensation, as though things done today occurred a week ago.
- Momentary loss of thought caused by sensation of tightness in brain. Loses constantly the thread of own speech. In conversation would occasionally stop, and on resuming remark on being unable to think of the right word to use.
- Perceives self as making wrong statements, out of not knowing what to say next; begins all right but does not know how to finish; weight on vertex, which seems to affect mind.[13]

In keeping with the respiratory aspect of Smell and also "go with the flow," we have:

- Intense itching in nose near its point, a need to rub all the time
- Very great burning in both nostrils when breathing through them
- Whole urethra feels sore, with a feeling as if something remained behind after urinating; in gleet

- Coldness of end of nose
- Entire loss of smell for several days
- Soreness of outer wing (inside) of left nostril
- Nasal catarrh, with continual running down the throat
- Sensation of action in bones of nose; obstruction at root of nose as if mucous membrane were hypertrophied (excessively bulky)
- Nose goes to sleep
- Nose is inflamed or swollen

Natrum muriaticum

Honoring the loss

All resources to the periphery	If I am good, no one gets hurt
Rejects hacksaw of grief	Prefers intimacy at arm's length
Impact of salt on metabolism	

Let us revisit a remedy discussed in the Inborn Toolkit section, Natrum muriaticum. A woman for whom this remedy made from sodium chloride, table salt, is beneficial might have been described as a young girl as having an emotionally sensitive nature. For our purposes this indicates enjoyment of poetry, a tendency to form powerful emotional attachments, a readiness to cry or laugh easily, and a capacity to be profoundly moved by significant events. At age twelve this girl suffered the loss of her mother, with whom she had enjoyed an especially strong bond.

Her grief proved difficult to process. Well into adulthood she is marked by diminished ability to cry (unless sobbing uncontrollably in private), accept consolation, or outwardly display emotion. She has perfectionist tendencies, a habit of smiling inappropriately when relating sad events, allergies, and insomnia due to distressing memories. Her mindset is that if she does nothing wrong then no one else will be hurt.

The Bible propounds a peril attending attachment to the past. It does so in its tale of Sodom and Gomorrah, where the wicked city of Sodom is about to be destroyed by God. Tasked with fleeing devastated Sodom, Lot's wife is warned by the angels not to look back at her former abode. The punishment reserved for her, one in keeping with our homeopathic interpretation of sodium chloride, is that Lot's wife, upon looking back, is transformed into a pillar of salt.

Unlike psychologists, homeopaths are not restricted to noting only mental and emotional symptoms. Specific physical symptoms can be included as well. Thus, headache or eye pain made worse from exposure to the sun, back pain ameliorated by strong pressure, a tendency to constipation or hemorrhoids, and cravings for salt and chocolate are included in our subject's profile.

For our subject, employing the hacksaw of grief to cut through the intensely experienced feeling of abandonment after the death of her mother is a nonstarter, as it would be perceived as an act of disloyalty to her mother. Compounding the girl's difficulty in allowing grieving to progress is a second idea: If her crying adequately expressed the depth of her grief, her tears would be never ending. In her suppressed state as a grown woman she retains a hot-button susceptibility to overriding sadness and melancholy. All that is needed for an episode of depression to be triggered is for the hot button to be pushed. She is triggered by almost any experience suggestive of loss. Our subject's emotional life is a dilemma summed up by the statement *I am desperate for intimacy but keep it at arm's length.*

Many caregivers would justifiably determine our subject to be clinically depressed. Homeopathic and dimensional reasoning lends further perspective to this diagnosis. To need Natrum muriaticum, meaning to be under the influence of sodium chloride, denotes a state of being self-contained, an idea familiar in regard to the relationship between excess salt intake and hypertension. Salt holds water in the cells, thereby increasing arterial pressure. We can compare the Nat mur subject to a besieged country that expends excessive resources defending its periphery. Although the country appears outwardly strong, within its borders it is tender and weak. Perhaps a means other than Natrum muriaticum can dispel our subject's need to overprotect the interior. Successful treatment via the remedy does the trick, prompting the taking up the hacksaw of grief so that her overattachment to the past can be cut. To experience the fullness of a present moment, to reclaim her orientation in time, is her due.

Natrum sulphuricum

I count for nothing

Melancholy

Suicidal

Worse from dampness

Mania

Skin ailments

Digestive system

Responsibility

Objectivity

Feels inconsequential

Head trauma

Individuals needing this grief remedy, also known as Glauber's salt, are deeply moved by music but emotionally self-contained. They are sensitive, but private with hurt feelings. Natrum sulphuricum people are responsible, melancholy, facts-oriented, and objective but also display the roller-coaster mania often labeled bipolar disorder. As it is but a short mental leap between the idea "I count for nothing" to "I might just as well not be here," risk of suicide within the remedy state is significant.

A major skin remedy, Natrum sulphuricum is indicated for sycotic outgrowths such as wartlike red lumps all over the body and eczema that is moist and oozing. Resulting from excessive production of catarrh or phlegm, their digestive disturbances engender a desire to be internally cleansed, evident from heightened satisfaction following complete bowel movements. The remedy is a prime complement of Thuja occidentalis, which expresses an anguished, self-recriminating, and inauthentic state that often serves to insulate the person from unbearable grief. Dispelling of the Thuja occidentalis layer, not surprisingly, prompts a grief-laden remedy state such as that associated with Natrum sulphuricum or Natrum muriaticum to surface.

Given how little conventional medicine has to offer people who have suffered one or more concussions, Natrum sulphuricum's prominence as a remedy for the lasting effects of head trauma is of immense importance. In the wake of concussion Arnica should immediately be given. If disorientation, vertigo, headache, or impaired cognition lingers, high-potency Natrum sulphuricum (or possibly another remedy, Cicuta virosa) is highly recommended.

Nux moschata

Life is unreal

Premature, not fully born	Drowsy/tired
Unsettled/excess privilege	Memory loss
Inappropriate smiling	Irregular menses

A notion that life is unreal is an existentialist trope. How much truth this contains is debatable. The Nux moschata state, in which life's unreality is actual, may shed light on the philosophical question. The remedy state's stupor, insensibility, and formidable need to sleep reflects or promotes a need to escape in the wake of some serious fright. In my experience the pattern originates early in life from a frightening loss or psychological neglect that may include an excess of caring or privilege, which conveys the message that the individual's world is artificial and unreal.

This nutmeg-derived remedy is the first to consider for narcolepsy. Sleepiness is a feature of almost all complaints. The individual appears dazed and forgetful. Though she is robotic in her actions, her state of mind is wondrous for its fitful, quickly switching moods. At one moment there is the deepest sorrow, then all at once frolicsome behavior, then a grave mien; then once again lighthearted. An individual in this state who is interrupted in a task or conversation forgets what the task or conversation was.

Older homeopathic materia texts speak of Nux moschata state's relevance for what were then called hysterical women. In updated terms this describes a loss of declarative memory (retention of information about facts or events over a significant period of time) and a retrograde amnesia (inability to recall past events) related to a problem within hippocampus brain function. Though speaking knowledgeably about the moment, this woman recalls nothing of the past.

Clairvoyance, prophesying, and predicting the future are also remedy features. On the physical plane we see excessive dryness of the tongue, mouth, lips, and throat. The individual is thirstless, and worse from cold damp weather, getting wet, and after a meal.

Sabina

Misbegotten

Uterine hemorrhage	Cysts, tumors, fig warts
Miscarriage susceptibility	Music penetrates and aggravates
Pain radiating from back to pubis	Internal heat
Pulsating blood	Duality of mind

Against her will a woman has conceived. Is there a more existential issue? Elaborating on the problem is a myth based on historical reality: a tale of the rape of the Sabine women, whose painful quandary the remedy Sabina encapsulates, the fallout from which it ameliorates.

Soon after the founding of Rome in the eighth century BCE a plan was hatched by Romulus, the founder and king of Rome, and his male followers to solve a problem: Since much of Rome's demographic then consisted of bandits, a sufficient number of civically oriented Roman men to defend the city was not at hand. This caused a concern for the declining population. With few women of reproductive age, there was a concern that the city might not survive. So as to guarantee a robust legacy for their city, a plan evolved whereby Sabine women from several neighboring towns would be "raped" (kidnapped) and forcibly wed to Roman men. According to the historian Livy in his famous fifteenth-century historical text, *Ab urbe condita* (From the founding of the city), some thirty women were abducted by the Romans during the festival of Neptune Equester.[14]

With the exception of one Sabine woman, Hersilia, who eventually became the wife of Romulus, the women were said to have all been virgins. Outraged, one of the neighboring kings invaded Roman territory and conflagration thereafter flared between the Sabines and the Romans. During a particularly heated conflict a remarkable thing happened: Anguished over the bloodshed and desperate to save both their fathers and their new husbands, the Sabine women threw themselves directly into the midst of the warring armies and implored them to stop fighting.

In non-homeopathic dosage the herb sabina is a well-known abortifacient. In homeopathic dosage Sabina addresses uterine hemorrhage and a miscarriage-inducing (especially in the third month) susceptibility to miscarriage that we see rooted in ambivalence concerning the fetus. At its most extreme the woman will pulsate from heated blood and experience pain radiating from the back to the pubis. A fascinating Sabina symptom is intolerance to music, which is experienced as penetrating and unnerving. Is it music's purity and generally unambiguous emotional import, so directly opposed to the woman's ambiguous feelings, that makes it intolerable? Or is it the tormenting knowledge that unambiguously pure vibrations, inaccessible to her, are reaching her unborn child?

Recent repeal of the *Roe v. Wade* ruling permitting abortion is likely to spur increased need for the Sabina remedy.

That Sabina is a sycotic remedy is evident from:

- Duality of the mind and identity *(How should I be oriented? To my husband or my father and brothers? Do I have a right to abort this being within me?)*
- Sabina's being a major remedy for gonorrhea for both men and women (also the presence of fig warts)
- The proliferation of skin and epithelial tissue symptoms, such as cysts, tumors, and warts

Samarium

Inside a bell jar

Lanthanide autonomy theme	Irregular menses
Lonely fight for freedom	Savior mindset
Heavy burden of a visionary	Mental suffocation
Self-imposed spiritual quest	Migraine headache

As Jan Scholten explains it, "Samarium's quality is heaviness. All the Lanthanides are heavy, but Samarium is extremely heavy. It's as if they carry the burden of the whole earth on their shoulders." In the face of all resistance and pain, they carry on. Samarium people are real builders for whom the pressure of a weighty mission instigates migraines.

Samarium, according to Scholten, "is the most pronounced migraine remedy of the Lanthanides."[15]

Underlying this heaviness is an excess of centeredness: The Lanthanide's thematic drive for autonomy has become a centripetal and isolating force. She exists in a bell jar for the self-reinforcing reason that in her visionary quest no one else can be relied upon to supply moral or spiritual guidance. Scholten points out the scope of symptoms emanating from this centripetal energy:

- Migraine
- Symptoms of the medial muscles of the eyes; glaucoma
- Lung ailments: granulomas, pneumoconiosis, bronchitis, pneumonia, tuberculosis
- Chest pressure, very heavy
- Liver pain, the pain spatially having the form of an old-fashioned key
- Liver problems: necrosis, fatty degeneration; spleen problems
- Colitis, diarrhea
- Kidney problems
- Male: ailments of the testis, epididymis, seminal vesicles, infertility
- Female: ailments of the ovaries, uterus; infertility, miscarriage; birth expulsion difficult
- Arthritis
- Blood: platelets, coagulation problems

Senega
Alienated

Easily offended	Inflammation of the pleura of lungs
Anxious/mortified	Bronchitis
Hasty respiration	Faint in open air

Senega, known as snakeroot, has domain over the mucous membranes, which makes it prominent for treating catarrhal symptoms of the respiratory tract, but also of the bladder. It is of use in complaints of the eyes and the pleura of the chest and circumscribed spots in the chest cavity after inflammation. The individual may feel faint when walking in open air. It is of use for sprains and for a sensation of trembling where the trembling is not visible.

Michal Yakir provides a window into the existential theme of this plant: alienation. The individual reacts with "sensitivity to everything that is 'other' to the person, which expresses itself physically through allergies and emotionally through temper tantrums and constant movement stemming from the inability to incorporate the emotions."[16]

The sense of "other" is reciprocal, meaning that not just the environment but the individual himself is other or alienated. As the child of Holocaust survivors living a seemingly undeserved normal life innocent of the torments my parents had encountered, I was subject to chronic coughs and bronchitis and was unaccountably over-reactive—a hothead. It was only after dosing myself with Senega that I acknowledged and then was able to release an ingrained sense of my "otherness." Liberation from alienation felt like I had rejoined the human race. As a bonus my respiratory ailments dissipated.

Sepia

Where am I in life?

Since hope is toxic, stagnate!	Misspeaks
The waters are muddied	"Natural" woman, loves dance
Indifference/apathy	

We revisit another remedy introduced in the Inborn Toolkit section. This is Sepia, and its name denotes its source—the ink of a sea creature, the cuttlefish. Ink's black color absorbs light, a quality that metaphorically, but also literally, accounts for Sepia's remedy picture, which like the event horizon of a black hole swallows up the light of life, namely hope. Like ink spilled on and blotting out portions of an important document, Sepia erodes clearly held distinctions critical to healthy Liver function. Its relation to light, blood function, and the Liver indicates that Sepia should be classified within the sense dimension of Sight. Due to the prominence of its disorientation features, which include feeling "lost" in life and misspeaking (the waters are muddied), it is positioned within sycosis and Smell.

The Sepia remedy state describes stagnation resulting from the effects of disappointment that is itself rooted in a blurring of distinction, such as when a depressed individual laments, "Even though my partner cheats on me, my partner still loves me."

Although not exclusively so, Sepia is largely a woman's remedy. On the physical plane, dysmenorrhea that is treatable with Sepia results from a profound stagnation that expresses itself in menstrual irregularity: The period may be late and scanty, early and profuse, or absent.

Traditional Chinese Medicine teaches that the Spleen is responsible for bolstering the organs and holding them in their rightful place; this function is deranged in the Sepia state. Commonly experienced within Sepia is a bearing-down sensation, as if everything inside is escaping from the vulva, and symptoms of uterine prolapse. Women having an affinity for its state are, to invoke the famous Aretha Franklin song, "natural women." They like to dance and enjoy nature; they are animated, affectionate, and invested in the idea that life progresses in a naturally forward-moving direction. When disappointment intrudes on their life path, symptoms of resentfulness, sarcasm, tearfulness, fatigue, and emotional indifference to a spouse or child crop up to serve as a bitter commentary on the natural state.

Other symptoms further illuminate the underlying problem. A person needing Sepia will be prone to nausea, acid reflux, or lack of appetite after taking only a few bites of food. Eruptions of the skin occur with healing crusts that prematurely flake off, thus causing the skin to heal twice. This symptom mirrors Sepia's sarcastic state of mind: *Sure, I'll make a half-hearted effort to heal, but that is the best I can manage.*

A Sepia woman generally is subject to flushes of heat and faintness, symptoms by now understandable as consequences of the stagnation of Liver chi. The tendency to misspeak expresses confusion, possibly arising from an unsatisfactory transition through one or another of life's developmental milestones. Further, troublesome experiences during puberty, early sexual events, marriage, childbirth, or menopause may increase resentment with each state she must say goodbye to—be it childhood innocence, puberty, loss of virginity, childlessness, or maternity—and may introduce confusion and uncertainty into her readiness to enter a succeeding developmental state.

Sepia's radical disjunct may be described as a natural state of hopefulness inviting its opposite, the bitter realization that hope itself is toxic. In the event that psychotherapy fails to cleanse hopefulness of its toxicity, it is fortunate that Sepia is available to enable restoration of hopefulness to its natural state.

Thuja occidentalis
An inauthentic life

Demolished self-esteem	Mental gymnastics
Self-deprecation	Warts from inner ugliness
Chameleon	No access to own self-interest

Let us deconstruct the existentialist notion of inauthenticity. The remedy Thuja occidentalis (made from arborvitae, recognizable as the tree of life) helps us do so. The Thuja occidentalis individual is an inauthentic person out of touch with his own self-interest. This individual may exhibit aspects of slavish conformism, artificial niceness, and falsity of self while harboring feelings of being unlovable with inner ugliness, hatred of the body, guilt, and shame. The famous self-deprecating joke of Groucho Marx—that he would not join a club that would have him as a member—embodies this idea.

The individual may also have a delusion of the soul having been separated from the body. The radical disjunct is that social acceptance of the false self confirms that the authentic self is unacceptable. The most striking physical symptoms of Thuja occidentalis relate to skin pathologies, particularly the appearance of odd or mushroom-shaped warts, as alluded to by sycosis's fig-wart disease nomenclature. A modern term for these warts, which are characteristic of HPV, is condylomata acuminata.

Not only the individual but a traumatized society also can lose its bearings and require Thuja occidentalis. Free-thinking, argumentative, and sensuous France was occupied by humorless, goose-stepping German soldiers during World War II. This was insulting to French honor and castrating to French identity. Jean Paul Sartre responded with an impenetrable, seven-hundred-page tome, *Being and Nothingness;* his argument that man is free ran perfectly counter to an opposite lesson imposed on French citizens who were compelled to squirm under the Nazi boot.

Sartre's existentialist depiction of social behavior as inauthentic and expressive of bad faith is itself inauthentic, since the term "bad faith" is an obfuscating term for dishonesty. Insofar as it serves only to camouflage a shattered national identity, Sartre's Marxist ideology can be taken with a grain of salt. The same can be said for situational ethics offered by existentialism to deflect attention from the country's humiliating Nazi collaboration. A generation later existentialist reasoning was to infect literary criticism in the contorted deconstructionist theory of Jacques Derrida, which delineated an ongoing process of questioning the accepted basis of meaning in language.

Fraught with conformism, fear, racism, and hypocrisy, post–World War II American society might have benefited from Thuja occidentalis in the drinking water. Here, the identity-shattering impetus was not Nazi occupation but shock. Following glorious victory in the war to end all wars and within the paradise of a booming economy, a monster had unexpectedly intruded, a new enemy capable of massive destruction. This was the Soviet Union with its thermonuclear arsenal.

Synchronically the iconic image of the era's fear, the mushroom cloud of a nuclear blast finds its parallel in a keynote symptom associated with the sycotic Thuja remedy: mushroom-shaped warts. The 1950s were guilty, secretive, and conformist years. Interestingly, the openness and self-liberation of the pursuant 1960s era embodied a closely linked sycotic nosode, Medorrhinum, that in clinical practice often follows Thuja occidentalis. There appeared in the 1950s an avatar for the era, an authentically inauthentic genius, Herman Kahn of the conservative Hudson Institute think tank.

Kahn blithely assured readers of his book, *On Thermonuclear War,* that nuclear war is survivable. He prognosticated that sufficient fallout shelters needed to be dug. Post-calamity, those emerging from underground would supposedly live comfortably within radioactive environs and amidst the neighboring corpses of millions. In the face of a threat of unfathomable calamity, mega-death master Kahn's dispassion strikes me as emotionally impoverished and inauthentic.

By way of response:

> *I will not carry myself down to die,*
> *When I go to my grave, my head will be high.*
> *Let me die in my footsteps before I go down under the*
> *ground.*
>
> BOB DYLAN,
"LET ME DIE IN MY FOOTSTEPS," 1962

In the late 1990s when invited to give a talk on homeopathy at the Kripalu Center for Yoga & Health, I presented a case involving Thuja occidentalis. The subject was a young man who worked as a car salesman and had sought me out for acupuncture for pain in his feet. Something about his appearance struck me as odd so I asked homeopathic questions. Perplexed as to my inquiries, he eventually related a matter he considered unrelated: He had persuaded his therapist to endorse his desire for a sex change. The odd look I noticed signified incompleteness of his hormonal regimen. I responded, "You feel you were born a woman in a man's body?" To my amazement he responded, "No, I'm attracted to women. What's the big deal?"

At this point I advised my Kripalu audience that I had no problem with lesbians, gay people, or what were then called transvestites (which I now know is a derogatory term). It was the nonchalance of the young man's quest to commence cross-dressing and transform into a lesbian in full view of a mainstream car-buying clientele that concerned me. His passion to undertake so momentous a change was for no better reason than "I'm unhappy, women seem happy, I'll become a woman." The roundabout reasoning struck me as contorted and evincing inability to access self-interest. Though an anticlimactic development, his response to the remedy bore me out. A few weeks after the consult he called me to say he was canceling the follow-up appointment. "Why?" I asked. "Oh," he said, "the treatment worked." His feet no longer hurt.

The Kripalu audience was wildly curious as to whether my patient went forward with the sex change. I told them I never found out and it was not my concern. What mattered to me was that regardless of the gender he ultimately chose, my client would thereafter be comfortable in his (or her) own skin. That he would desist with his mental gymnastics, gain access to his self-interest, and live an authentic life was my hope.

The majority of the audience, made up largely of therapists, was intrigued to learn that despite having no agenda—in fact *because* it was agenda-less—homeopathy worked. But in a foreshadowing of the encompassing, self-righteous intolerance of gender identity discourse today (2023), my relating of the case struck a nerve with a subset of the audience then on retreat at Kripalu. This contingent's leader was incredulous that for the homeopath nothing is off limits. I explained how turning a deaf ear to the young man's gender exploration would have led to my choosing an ineffective remedy. She remained adamant that my investigation was outrageous. During our email exchange I inquired how the normal practice of homeopathy, in which judgments are not made and behavioral recommendations never offered, can possibly be dangerous. This was beside the point, she insisted. I must have had an agenda, and a sinister one at that. I needed to be canceled.

The CEO, who had personally invited me to the center, apologized for the embarrassing turn of events. But then, as he explained, the aggrieved contingent was a sizable presence at Kripalu, so he had no choice but to accede to their demand. I was branded a dangerous person and banned from ever presenting at Kripalu again.

Masked Depression and
Thuja occidentalis

A teenage boy was brought to me who had convinced himself that he was a robot. He had encountered a biology class teaching about Darwinism suggesting that random, environmentally induced characteristics of an organism overrode the organism's—or an individual's—free will. Obsessed with the idea that "he" could not possess personhood, he had deduced that he was a robot. Certitude that he had no free will defeated several therapists who tried to overthrow his delusion. I told him that since I'd treated numerous robots in the past, he posed me no problem. My prescription was Thuja occidentalis.

About six weeks after a patient has taken a constitutional dose of Thuja occidentalis the more obvious symptoms abate. A remedy embodying whatever underlying trauma the Thuja occidentalis layer has been insulating then emerges. This is what happened with my robot patient. At the follow-up, by his own admission he was no longer a robot. Instead he now presented as a depressed but more authentic teenager. Strong enough now in the wake of Thuja occidentalis to confront underlying trauma, his condition called for a complementary remedy for grief and depression. This was the remedy Natrum sulphuricum, which I then prescribed to good effect.

Iscador (fermented Viscum album)
Caught between two worlds

Suspended between alternate realities	Abstraction of mind
Cancer via heredity	Epilepsy
Environmental impact	Tearing pains
Impaired immunity	

Our discussion of Viscum album will provide the remarkable example of existential disorientation's implication in serious illness: the etiology of cancer of the breast and large intestine rooted in disorientation occurring at the genetic level.

Viscum album is derived from tincture made of the fresh berries and leaves of the parasitic mistletoe plant. The books speak of its use for a sensation that one is about to topple; a glow rising from the feet to the head as if it were on fire; paralysis of every muscle, except those of the eye; inability to speak or swallow; spectral illusions; insensibility; and stupor. It is used to lower high blood pressure and for rheumatic complaints and sciatica, epilepsy, chorea, metrorrhagia, asthma deafness from a rheumatic cause, and spinal pains due to uterine causes. According to Madeline Evans, it addresses karmic issues that undermine immunity and predispose cancer and epilepsy.[17]

The individual in need of Viscum album is much in touch with the interplay between scripted destiny (immunity) and toxic exposure. This serves to enlarge a disoriented awareness of being caught between two worlds, a sense that the phenomenon of an epileptic seizure both reflects and promotes.

Viscum album's mental symptoms denote this sense of being caught between two worlds. This is evident in a delusion of the body being lighter than air, seeing figures during half sleep, feeling as if in a dream, having frightful thoughts on waking at night, and experiencing time as passing too quickly.

Anthroposophical medicine offers a terrain-based description of the fermented version of this medicine. Called Iscador, its scope of action affects the delicate balance between the organism and the environment, as well as within the organism maintaining homeostasis in the face of toxic exposure. Mistletoe therapy is increasingly recognized as a viable option for cancer. It contains several compounds, including lectins, that augment immune defense while ameliorating the negative effects of cancer treatments.[18]

The Paulina Medical Clinic in Chicago and European doctors have been using homeopathic potencies of the plant to treat cancer with some success.[19]

The remedy figures into treatment of the precancerous state where the effects one can see are in the depressed, prematurely aging patients with insufficient hormonal and enzymatic functions who blossom into new life. Another important sphere of action is the postoperative prevention of recurrences of a carcinoma whereby daily injections of Iscador for several weeks energize resistance.

CANCER OF THE BREAST AND LARGE INTESTINE: FRAMESHIFT MUTATIONS

When we characterize a particular trait or disease as genetic, we generally mean that its emergence is preordained. Expressing a biochemical disorder, or glitch, the genetic trait or disease lies outside our ordinary sphere of influence. What so frightens people about cancer is therefore its uncontrollability. A mechanism is seen as going haywire in the program according to which cells normally divide and cease dividing. Previously typical cells begin to multiply rapidly and invasively in a process that nerve and hormonal action are at a loss to control.

Not all the news is bleak. It is now clear that an important distinction exists between our genetic design, or genotype, and healthful or unhealthful gene expression, or phenotype. The phenotype may be modified by lifestyle as well as by activating the mind-body connection.

Disorientation at the Genetic Level

Centeredness opposes disorientation even at the genetic level. Both the colon and breasts are vulnerable to orientation-related issues because they are components of the large intestines and chest, anatomic regions associated with the sense dimension of Smell. Within their tissue, malignancies notable for the chaos that governs cell replication can arise. Forms of these cancers result from a particularly devastating type of mutation known as a frameshift, which occurs at the genetic level.

Genetic replication can be likened to a linguistic process that requires a context of meaning to be sustained. When disorientation manifests at the linguistic level, the sounds of words cease to express their proper meanings; like a worn-out fabric, the context of our mental associations has fallen apart. A nucleotide equals a frame that is being read. In terms of a linguistic analogy, the frame equals the context of meaning. During gene replication, messenger RNA, using the DNA as a template, copies a series of instructions for protein synthesis. The expression of these instructions is virtually a prose sentence in which codons (a specific sequence of three DNA bases within a gene, responsible for directing the synthesis of amino acid molecules possessing highly specific molecular structures that are vital for the formation of proteins) are the constituent words. The nucleotides themselves may be thought of as syllables.

In a single nucleotide polymorphism, substitution of an incorrect nucleotide during transcription of DNA bases in the production of messenger RNA generally alters only a single triplet group. Leaving the remaining sequence of codons unaltered, this is a nonsense mutation, the equivalent of which is writing a set of instructions for the manufacture of a defective shoe that, once it leaves the assembly line, is found to lack a specific feature, such as eye holes for laces. In the much more serious *missence* mutation known as a frameshift, the bases in an entire sequence of codons within a molecule of messenger RNA following the deletion (or addition) of a single nucleotide frame-shift forward or backward. This leaves the following sequence of bases scrambled. An unusual degree of disorganization to the gene packet involving genetic replication results. A frameshift mutation is thus a nonsense mutation leaving nothing but chaos in its wake. It is the equivalent of a set of shoe manufacturing instructions that somewhere in the middle of the paragraph degenerates into total nonsense. When the instructions are precisely followed an object unrecognizable as a shoe rolls off the assembly line. Contorted protein synthesis due to a frameshift mutation almost always results in dysfunction ranging from mild abnormality to malignancy.

The Potent Sense Dimension of
Smell Mutagen Acridine

The environmental toxin acridine, a hydrocarbon compound that is a by-product of coal combustion used in the manufacture of dyes, biological stains, and antibacterial agents, is a mutagen and the most acrid gas known. Positively charged acridine dyes bind directly to the DNA; they sandwich themselves between stacked base pairs of DNA, inserting or deleting one base pair in DNA, resulting in frameshift mutations.

The TP53 gene provides instructions for making a protein called tumor protein p53 (or transformation-related protein 53). This protein acts as a tumor suppressor, which means that it regulates cell division by keeping cells from growing and dividing (proliferating) too fast or in an uncontrolled way. Because the protein p53 is essential for regulating DNA repair and cell division, it has been nicknamed the "guardian of the genome." Research shows that TP53 mutations that result in loss of transcriptional activity are commonly found in numerous types of cancer.[20] Research shows they are frequently found in non–small cell lung cancer.[21]

A remedy of importance is Lapis albus, indicated for epithelioma, the pre-ulcerative stage of carcinoma, and cancers of the breast as well as of the glands and uterus, when burning and stinging pains denote the toxic effect of acridine. Meat aversion within the remedy picture implicates acridine-related umami smell associated with cooked meat. Justifiably, Lapis albus's importance is cited in A. U. Ramakrishnan's plussing protocol (a method of increasing the potency of a remedy by systematically diluting and shaking it) for cancer of the breast.[22]

Various therapeutic practices can help promote health within the sense dimension of Smell.

Smell Dimension Health Promotion Practices

- Develop a strategic capability.
- Minimize scent pollution.

- Nurture the mother of Smell, Taste: Identify and accept genuine challenges.
- Meditate; harmonize the breath.
- Process grief, then move on.
- Nurture family ties.

4

Can the boundary between life and death be abided?

Syphilitic Miasm • Hearing • Water Phase •
Fear • Kidneys–Urinary Bladder

Is there life after death? If there is no life after death, why not gratify my every want and wish? If what I do in this life impacts my descendants, how can I improve my legacy? My fingers clench around the pliers of fear; do I let go and hurtle forward? Or hold tight and stay put? Such questions lie at the core of the syphilitic miasm and underlie what I have termed the sense dimension of Hearing.

THE SYPHILITIC MIASM AND
THE SENSE DIMENSION OF HEARING

As Samuel Hahnemann observed, when the acute sexually transmitted disease syphilis and its primary manifestations, chancre and bubo (lymph swelling), are suppressed by some violent local treatments, the venereal miasm syphilis emerges. For this reason it is also called the "chancre disease." The mode of infection described in the literature as impure coition reflects a conjunction of poor hygiene, undue friction in a tender center of nerve-rich tissue, and the stress of guilt and secrecy accompanying illicit sexual behavior.

Once the syphilitic miasm gains a foothold it ceases to be local and

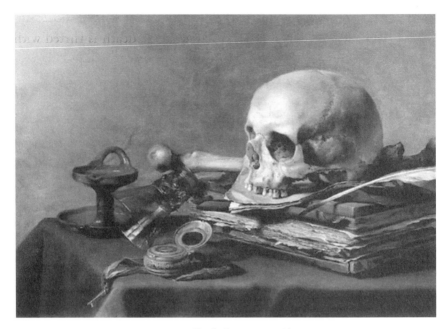

Vanitas Still Life by Pieter Claesz

becomes a general dynamic. From this point on wiping, cleansing, corroding, and cauterizing of the infected spot will be in vain. Here in the secondary stage conventional suppressive care compels the organism to supplant the dessicated chancre with a more painful eruption, namely the bubo. Other signs of the secondary state include fever of usually less than 101°F; sore throat; a vague feeling of weakness or discomfort throughout the body; weight loss; patchy hair loss, especially in the eyebrows, eyelashes, and scalp hair; and swelling of the lymph nodes. Nervous system symptoms can include neck stiffness, headaches, irritability, paralysis, unequal reflexes, and irregular pupils.[1]

The most destructive phase, the tertiary stage may begin as early as one year after infection and thereafter. Its complications include gummata, large sores inside the body or on the skin; cardiovascular syphilis, which affects the heart and blood vessels; and neurosyphilis, which affects the nervous system. In the nineteenth and early twentieth century this was called general paresis, also known as general paralysis of the insane (GPI). This denoted paralytic dementia that would include depression, mania, psychosis, personality changes, delirium, dementia, and suicidality.

Is the boundary between life and death to be abided? In the suicidality a back-and-forth game can be played where death is flirted with nonchalantly: *If the phone rings in the next five minutes I won't do it. If it doesn't then I will.* Or *I'll flip a coin: Heads I do it, tails I don't.*

The Sense Dimension of Hearing

Wuxing phase: Water
Emotion: Fear
Organ: Kidneys–Urinary Bladder
Theme: Consolidation vs. entropy

This is a complex and intricate dimension. Reflecting fluid metabolism and reproductive function and what is known as the Water phase in TCM, the sense dimension of Hearing concerns a core opposition between healthful consolidation and pathological entropy.

Hearing is the ability to interpret audible sound, based on the collection and transformation of fluctuations in pressure. The cognitive aspect of hearing—the selective act of listening—has no equivalent among the other four senses. Within the cacophony of surrounding sound we attend to what interests us and turn a deaf ear to all else. Hearing requires us to discriminate between what we permit to pass through and what we do not. Ability to shift attention within sound may result from a distinct neurological feature: As opposed to other sensory pathways, the auditory pathway is bilateral. Sensory fibers issuing from each of the two auditory cochlea within the inner ear are both crossed and uncrossed. Each cochlea is represented in both hemispheres of the brain. Even if we were deaf in one ear our hearing would remain stereophonic.

Our inner-ear mechanism is an arrangement of intricate tubing filled with fluid. It has many similarities with a system of hair and canals found in fish; archlike tissues found in the middle ear resemble gill-like slits. The human middle ear appears to have evolved from the first two arches (and the neck structure containing them). This system, known as the lateral-line canal, allows fish while swimming to detect variations in water pressure and the presence of moving objects such as predators. Our modern hearing sense is consequently an elaboration on the kinesthetic awareness of fish moving about in water. In order to make the transmission of sound more efficient, the external auditory canal connecting the outer ear and the eardrum is lined by a combination of epithelial and periosteum tissue. A pervasive theme of Water involves energetic interplay within the body between epithelial and osseous (bone or periosteum) tissue.

TCM's existential notion of Water is an amphitheater where sex-and-death dramas written or celebrated by luminaries are staged. The list includes philosophers, the originators of the Greek myths, and the tragic playwrights Sophocles, Euripedes, O'Neill, and Ibsen as well as scientists of the mind such as Sigmund Freud. Also included is the postulator of a conflict between eros, the life instinct, and thanatos, the death instinct, Hungarian psychoanalyst Sándor Ferenczi.

WATER PHASE AND TRADITIONAL CHINESE MEDICINE

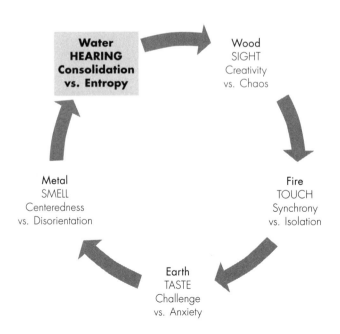

Traditional Chinese Medicine presents the season of winter as pertaining to the phase of Water. This denotes depths below the surface. The organ pairs highlighted during winter are the Kidneys and Urinary Bladder, whose meridian pathways are chief purveyors of the chi or life force of our being. The emotion associated with Water is fear, encountered earlier in the pliers of fear section of the Inborn Toolkit.

CONSOLIDATION VERSUS ENTROPY

That for which we have no use would be toxic if retained, meaning in service to entropy. Therefore, it is discarded. That which is valued not only is retained but permanently secured, and thus the subject of consolidation. This idea is at play within TCM's elaboration of the Water domain, said to rule the Kidneys and Urinary Bladder, which in Chinese medicine include the bones, epithelium, and much of reproductive function.

- Kidney function involves directing impure fluid to the Urinary Bladder to be excreted, while pure fluid is retained and consolidated as essence.
- Though the epithelium is soft and moist while the bones are dry and hard, both serve Water due to their function as boundaries between cells and tissue. Comprising the foundation of our structural integrity, a bastion against entropic collapse and the body's most durable tissue, able to survive its demise, the bones epitomize Hearing-dimension consolidation.
- The *yuan* or original chi residing within the Kidneys represents genetic information consolidated as part of the miasma (homeopathic view) within our legacy (TCM view) or genome (biomedical view). Yuan can also be viewed as conveying miasma to the *hun,* or ethereal soul (comparable to Jung's notion of the collective unconscious), via our parents and ancestors. These are now consolidated within the Kidneys of the newborn child.
- Consolidation: Healthful mitochondria from the mother are established within the fetus. Kidney yang projects the will and

purpose-laden hun into the body at birth, only to extract and eject it back to its universal source at death. A well-adjusted child, having successfully resolved centeredness versus disorientation, is prepared for the onerous lifetime demands of hearing and acquiescing to his life mission—in other words, accessing his hun and serving his will.

- Entropy: Problematic resolution of consolidation versus entropy may be due to dysfunctional resolution of centeredness versus disorientation. Or it may reflect perpetuation of an unimproved-upon or even worsened legacy. In *The Spell of the Sensuous* David Abram explores the sense of hearing via phenomenological investigation of the voice and nature.[2] A review by Bill McKibben quoted on the cover captures the book's wonders and relevance to the dimension of Hearing: "Manages almost magically to stir in us long-lost memory: deep in our bones, in our blood, in the air we breathe, we know the world lives and speaks to us . . . shows that it is possible to reawaken the animistic dimension of perception and feeling without renouncing rationality and intellectual analysis."

It is said within TCM that congenital illness manifests within the Kidney yang. Other than a random occurrence, the presence of congenital illness represents information that, through consolidation (compression into an inheritable "coded" form), gained immortality. What might that information be and how does it come to be consolidated?

Jing and the Consolidation (Inheritance) of Stress

Jing is an essential energy stored within the Kidneys. When circulating throughout the body it is known as yuan, which translates as reproductive essence—inborn, genuine, or original chi. Jing issues mainly from the congenital essence of life (yet another form of chi stored in the Kidneys) but also is supplemented and nourished by the acquired essence of life that is produced by the metabolic efforts of the Spleen and Stomach. Although it also receives impetus from an unlimited supply of Kidney yang, jing is neither immortal nor infinite.

When we are run-down or depressed as a result of stress, jing's contraction (or, under more serious conditions, depletion) in mental, emotional, and physical terms undermines us. Jing is, in fact, a precious and finite substance whose conservation we should heed. Jing supports the Kidney yin's ability to supply epithelial moisture and general fluid function throughout the body. It possesses a power to motivate the vital activities of the body without which normal development, growth, and healing do not occur. Depletion of jing prompts lassitude, vertigo, debility, and susceptibility to illness. Therapeutic recourses such as acupuncture and herbal treatments owe their effectiveness to their ability to conserve and protect jing.

Within ancient Chinese texts, although sex is an equal and harmonious libido exchange equally benefiting both partners, excessive sexual activity depletes chi essence and blood in men. The material part of chi essence in the Kidneys making up the semen is then excreted from the body. TCM and the syphilitic miasm teach that excessive sexual activity should be avoided because seminal fluid is a precious chi essence. Its exhaustion is depleting and life shortening.

Due to its origination in the congenital essence of life, it sometimes happens that jing is congenitally of weak quality. Depending on the severity of jing deficiency, the reproductive organs may be undeveloped, undersized, or inoperative. The onset and regularity of puberty may be affected, as well as the production of gametes in a female and sperm in a male. This constitutional deficiency may prevent fertility and hamstring the interventions of artificial reproductive technology.

Situations of enduring stress, such as a severe and lasting encounter with a pathogen, cannot be indefinitely withstood. There exists a point beyond which even emergency resources are no longer available. It is at such a point that trauma and concern long borne by an overburdened jing is permitted to shift over and become imprinted upon the jing's more powerful partner, a suddenly informed and activated Kidney yang. When miasmatic symptoms erupt in a descendant one or more generations later, these are in effect the reverberating plaints of jing.

Although the concept of jing is missing from conventional medicine as well as homeopathy, its acceptance as a theoretical concept carries practical benefits. Jing should be thought of whenever dietary and nutritional changes are warranted. Entropic features of an individual or child within whom jing's complaints reverberate include savantism, autism, and behaviors and symptoms reflecting a legacy of drug abuse or alcoholism. Though by definition each of the miasms transmits inherited features, it is the syphilitic miasm in particular that consolidates deficiencies such as genetic mutations, organ deformities, and susceptibility to autoimmunity and coinfection.

The Syphilitic Miasm's Existential Themes
- Everything circles back to nothingness
- "Endless foreplay" circular thinking
- Death denied: materialism, profligacy
- Death accommodated: securing of legacy, community, well-being
- To sin or not to sin
- Redemption

TREATMENTS AND EXPECTATIONS

Remedies manifesting subcategories of *Can the boundary between life and death be abided?*

Adamas	Mercurius (vivus or solubilis)
Argentum metallicum	Petroleum raffinatum
Aurum metallicum	Syphilinum
Conium maculatum	Thulium
Fluoricum acidum	

Adamas (diamond trituration and untriturated immersion)

Loss of faith

Abuse	Loss of precious possession
Blackness	Sharp pains
Discouraged	Suicidal
Depressed	Weakness

Created deep in the earth from tremendously pressurized carbon, the gemstone diamond evinces a dire polarity: unimaginable value opposed by the nadir of worthlessness. Diamond associates with the adjective "adamantine," meaning unbreakable, impenetrable, impregnable. The Greek *adamas* denotes "unyielding, invincible."

Caught in its grip, the individual needing Diamond dances on a knife-edge between supreme accomplishment and uselessness. The elder version of the remedy, made from a trituration of Diamond, comes into play for deep discouragement. This is expressed via resentment, anger provoked by words or even gestures, irritability and taciturnity, and aversion to company. Its younger cousin, a remedy derived from an immersion of the whole substance, should be evoked when an amplified version of discouragement—complete loss of faith and hope to the point of suicidality—comes to the fore. Abuse, dreadful experiences, and the loss of a child or an irreplaceable possession is a gateway to the remedy state. A personal encounter with the remedy state occurred when I briefly lost my computer at an airport. The following forty-eight hours, before the computer was found, were the worst two days of my life.

Peter Tumminello, a sensitive prover with vast experience and the first person to prove Diamond immersion, reported that the medicine took him frighteningly close to suicide. In this case loss of faith in homeopathy, to which he was deeply committed, was at cause. On the positive side, an Adamas individual will have a sharp intellect.

Argentum metallicum

Is my legacy secure?

Loquacity/loss of voice	Reproduction/*cojones*
Creativity/"calling"	Electrical sensation
Prostration/serenity	Silver lining/silver spoon

Argentum metallicum, made from silver, has domain over the larynx. The remedy state's symptoms appear slowly, with a progressive loss of control over mind and body. The loss of mental power is insidious, as first there is talkativeness but then disinclination to speak in social circumstances. Early materia medica books speak of the individual being worse while speaking, while singing, or after mental strain. Respiratory symptoms described include hoarseness and aphonia (loss of all but whispered speech) that is aggravated from use of the voice. Argentum metallicum is a primary remedy for total loss of voice in professional singers. The upper limbs can feel powerless or the individual can suffer from writer's cramps. Peculiar symptoms that bring this remedy to mind include electrical sensations and a sense of serenity.

Silver is a precious metal, but care is taken so that, like a personal legacy, it does not tarnish. That its value requires upkeep is reflected in Jan Scholten's *Homeopathy and the Elements,* where Argentum metallicum's central position in the seventh row of the periodic table pertains to creativity and accomplishment. The remedy's essential idea concerns holding on to a successful position: "Their beautiful creations in the past have caused them to have high expectations of the future. Their parents, friends, the general public, everyone expects them to continue their successes. But they are afraid they might not be as good as they used to be, that they might not be able to perform as well as they did that time."[3]

Argentum metallicum personifies the need to consolidate in the face of entropy, as in looking to posterity, securing one's legacy in the wake of accomplishment. The remedy's relation to legacy is expressed idiomatically as when referring to a child of privilege as having been born with a silver spoon in his mouth. The relation of oratory to silver is expressed in saying someone "has a silver tongue."

An avatar of this remedy is Winston Churchill, a great orator with unparalleled mastery over his voice. Churchill was also a painter. The central trauma of his life is that Great Britain's loss of India, crown jewel of the British empire, on his watch undermined his and his country's legacy. Idiomatic support for Argentum metallicum's relevance to fertility issues is found in the testicles being referred to as crown jewels. They are the repository of a man's courage, potency, and, ultimately, legacy.

Aurum metallicum

Do my works please God?

Deep personal responsibility	Critical and self-critical
Depression/suicidality	Sensation of one's bones
Heartbreak/heart ailments	Moaning/praying

Aurum is made from gold. People needing this remedy already are or need to be "good as gold."

Moses, the Proving Master

As reported in Exodus 32, Moses took the golden calf, the false idol the Israelites had made, burned it in the fire, ground it to powder, and made the children of Israel drink of it. In doing so Moses unwittingly acted as homeopathic "proving master." When the Israelites consumed the diluted gold their behavior became more pleasing to God. The low potency but energized form of Aurum made the lesson stick.

The depressive despair Aurum metallicum so famously treats is usually rooted in the individual's having experienced heartbreak or devastating loss. By way of compensation he seeks to achieve synchrony with the highest realm of spirit, God. The means of doing so include high-level achievement, prayer, and other forms of spiritual practice to stave off entropy. The psychological profile is one who takes on huge responsibility.

Physical manifestations include cardiac symptoms, high blood pressure, angina, palpitations, and pain described as issuing from deep in the bones (the most consolidated tissue in the body). The radical disjunct pertains to a sense of self-worth that is linked to impossibly high standards. Self-worth must be proven through achievements that are never sufficient. The manic redoubling of efforts to achieve produces only exhaustion and greater despair, thereby establishing inherent worthlessness.

Predisposition to depression is attributed in homeopathy to the syphilitic miasm, whose equivalent within Traditional Chinese Medicine involves congenital disease features being imprinted onto the Kidney yang. Symptoms of the syphilitic miasm include an unusual sense of struggle, intractable circular reasoning, and strong sexuality, all of which also pertain to the remedy Syphilinum that I will discuss shortly.

Conium maculatum

The walls close in on me

Life's "juices" dry up	Emotionally difficult/dementia
Induration	Ascending paralysis
Cancer	Worse from excitement
The "Aconite of old age"	Jaded or resigned to fate
Terminated sex life	

There exists that instant when, from fear, our defense system suddenly weakens and an acute ailment is invited. If in this brief moment a dose of the remedy Aconitum napellus is taken, the onset can be derailed. Conium maculatum, made from poison hemlock, is called the Aconitum napellus of old age. When an interval in time crops up during which one feels suddenly old, a dose of Conium maculatum also scotches the deal.

Gateways to the Conium maculatum state include sudden loss of one's sex life, a crushing reversal of fortune, reaching a dreaded milestone birthday such as forty or fifty, or a last-straw disappointment. The life juices dry up, indurations (hard lumps) appear in the muscle tissue, paralysis ascends from the feet up through the legs, the limbs atrophy, a cancer may develop. On the mental/emotional plane is anger along with a feeling that the world is shrinking and the walls are closing in, creating a kind of claustrophobia. The radical disjunct is that an otherwise exciting development in life is perceived as a depressing development. A sense of resignation to one's plight ensues.

Recognizing that he would no longer be permitted to expand his students' horizons, and accepting the authorities' view that he had corrupted the youth of Athens, Socrates resigned himself to his fate and drank poison hemlock without complaint.

Case Study

A Child Needing Conium maculatum

Surprisingly, the Conium maculatum state's existential issue can arise in a child. It has been my honor to treat a young Down syndrome girl on my caseload, and whenever she becomes ill, it greatly illuminates the theme of the remedy I discern she needs. After "Minnie" responded well to Plumbum metallicum, prescribed to address a constipated and fearful state when she would stomp heavily around the room, she was brought to my office no longer fearful but bossy, a know-it-all, and with a jaded attitude in regard to newly gained freedom in place of her former fear.

Notes from a Session Following Dosage with Conium maculatum

Became positive, could focus on school . . . a tiny step back . . . she gets stuck . . . and you can talk to her about it . . . will initially resist . . . but you can talk to her. Because we constantly tell her what to do . . . she is doing that with her friends . . . telling the rules to her friends . . . like she wants to control other people's choices . . . Bossy, clinging to her certitudes. Wants to boss other, as in, It's my turn now to do this.

Much more tired . . . waking much later . . . wakes up groggy . . .

Roaming about everywhere at night, cannot settle into one position.

Looking forward to becoming a grown-up at middle school . . .

So now I'm a big girl, I can walk to school (things she had not done). Like she has given herself permission to be grown up.

Very tired in the evening, gets glassy eyed. Bravely went on a zip line during visit to a reservation.

Mother reports that somehow it is all wearing on Minnie. Like a know-it-all, the child will go and report all the "rules" to her younger brother.

Now experimenting with new foods . . . into carbs . . . chocolate. Apologizing a lot.

Had a bit of a cough but that came and went quickly.

Resisted going to her own school graduation ceremony. Going on her tippy-toes a bit. Mom suggests she may be dizzy. (Note: Conium maculatum is a very dizzy remedy.)

My conjecture is that the dizziness expresses confusion attending her switching to a more advanced level of schooling. With the higher ceiling of possibilities, Minnie must start at an entry level where she will feel inadequate. Whether Minnie's choices should reflect wider or narrower possibilities presents her with a dizzying conundrum.

I reference for the mother the famous Peggy Lee song, "Is That All There Is?" With regard to Minnie she agrees, saying, "Yeah, freedom: Is that all there is?"

The Conium maculatum went well. At our next session the pendulum swung in its opposite direction, with Minnie presenting what I determined to be Valeriana officinalis, featuring the opposite of jadedness—hypersensitivity—and an exaggerated display of what it looked like to be a grown-up.

Fluoricum acidum

Nothing counts other than the present

Ogling/libertarian	Immediate gratification
Materialism/spice of life	Relationship doomed
Buoyancy/poor focus	You're fired!

The boundary between life and death can be abided either through commitment to a spiritual path, according to which an enduring soul transitions to a higher plane of existence, or through denial of death, with the entropy of afterlife emptiness countered by the embrace of a materialistically driven existence on earth.

People needing Fluoricum acidum belong to the second category. According to master homeopath Rajan Sankaran, a materia medica of the Fluoricum acidum remedy describes the following (a perfect example of which would be former president Donald Trump):

- Glamour. The individual is drawn to glamour, will push anything and anyone aside in an all-absorbing desire to shine and glitter. Looking to be the big macho guy for everybody to look up to, this individual draws attention with a big car and high position, is ambitious, and wants to climb high and earn lots of money.
- Tendency to form superficial relationships. Fluorine is the lightest, the most active and reactive, forming and breaking relationships very quickly. This can be seen in the symptomatology of Fluoricum acidum. The remedy state is flirtatious; it has many acquaintances but no deep relationship. The term "buoyancy" has been used to describe it. The word is derived from that of the buoy, a conical object that floats on the surface of the ocean and never sinks or reaches any depth. The feeling of being in a fluorine state is abnormal for a human being, at any time.
- Immorality. Aversion to responsibility, sexual desire increased, attracted to strangers, and increased energy. A naive psychopath, prone to serious gambling.
- Delusions about servants he must eliminate. In other words, "You're fired!" Fluoricum acidum is the only remedy in this rubric.
- Mental buoyancy
- Compulsion to ignore taboos
- Isolation and narcissism
- Demand for sexual experience
- Dependency on property
- Ruthlessness

Illness Susceptibility in
Fluoricum acidum

Fluoricum acidum comes into play with regard to ailments of the bones, mucous membranes, and epithelium; complaints of old age and premature old age; sexual exhaustion; weak constitution; sallow skin; and emaciation.

Donald Trump's Handshake Phobia and
Obsession with Building a Wall

These well-known Trump traits reflect a germophobia feature pertaining to the syphilitic miasm to which Fluoricum acidum belongs. Homeopathy's foundational notion of the syphilitic miasm is Hearing's core conundrum inflamed to the point of consolidating syphilis's influence within familial legacy. The remedy Donald Trump needs, Fluoricum acidum, showcases a mentally buoyant, ruthless, and transgressive strain of the syphilitic miasm. Trump's inherited legacy displays the dilemma of an overcompensating outsider. Congenital difficulty accepting entropy draws him and those within his genetic line toward consolidating reliance on defensive structures such as walls (also projecting the syphilitic miasm's sense of separateness from others), materiality, and "time-compressed" pleasures such as sex. This is the remedy Fluoricum acidum.

Aurum fluoratum,
a Nuanced Alternative

Homeopath and author Pierre Fontaine (*One Heart, One Mind*) has suggested a nuanced alternative, Aurum fluoratum. The Aurum part, a syphilitic grief remedy on its own terms, speaks to Trump's grief over the loss of his older brother. It also fits with the way Trump takes good care of those in his charge (unless he is suddenly, as per the indicated Fluoricum acidum delusion, compelled to fire one of his stewards). The slogan "Make America Great Again" represents as an excess of responsibility, in keeping with Aurum.

Mercurius (vivus or solubilis)

Enemies everywhere

The world is a dangerous place	Mercurial regarding weather
Anarchist/troublemaker	Changeable temperament
Quick communicator/precocious	Grips tightly the pliers of fear
Emotionally closed	

In the 1800s in Europe, when mercury was used in manufacturing to cure hat felt, a form of mercury called mercurous nitrate was used. Having inhaled mercury vapors, many hatmakers developed neurological symptoms of mercury poisoning, which is how the expression "mad as a hatter" came into parlance. Thus, the remedy Mercurius (vivus or solubilis, the two being interchangeable) is of great value in the treatment of madness, especially of paranoid fear (in the grip of the pliers). Paranoia fueled by circular thinking on the mental plane and nerve tissue destruction on the physical plane betray the miasm's presence. For this we can blame past medical history during which syphilitic mercury's application in treating the actual disease syphilis was both extensive and excessive.

The derivation of the word "quack" reflects mercurial madness. The term was first and justifiably applied to medical doctors guilty of prescribing high levels of the toxic metal mercury for syphilis and also for a wide range of other ailments. In ancient times mercury was called quicksilver and so doctors routinely giving mercury to their patients became known as "quickers." In common usage the term was shortened to "quick." Then as patients underwent neurological decline and quickly expired, this word morphed into "quack."[4]

The task of cleaning up the mess left by allopathic (non-homeopathic) physicians thus fell to their homeopathic colleagues. Perhaps so as to deflect from the unpleasant history of quackery, mainstream apologists speculate that the Dutch word "kwakzalver" (seller of nostrums) is at the root of "quack." It can also be argued that the word contains "kwakken" (to impulsively fling an object), as in heedlessly flinging a worthless remedy at a sick individual.[5]

A clinical hallmark of mercury poisoning is, in fact, mercuriality, meaning changeability and impulsivity. It is likelier that the word "kwakzalver" is derived from "quicksilver," a name for mercury that has been used since the twelfth century.

As in Greek mythology Mercury is the god of communication, so is the Mercurius vivus patient an excellent communicator. Such an individual is also mercurial in being emotionally changeable and sensitive to changes in atmospheric pressure (which is why mercury is used in barometers). Communication skill notwithstanding, the Mercurius vivus individual is emotionally closed to the point of being virtually unknowable as a person. I suspect that such emotional suppression reflects a deluded notion that to mentally entertain a possibility guarantees that the possibility will actually occur (thus, be emotionally felt). So then if the emotionally charged possibility is dire, squashing it is necessary. When a possibility is positive the thought gains the status of a prophecy and merits being excitedly expressed.

The remedy state includes tremor, weakness of memory, indecent or anarchic behavior, peculiar notions about food, dullness of the eyes and staring, and suspicion and distrustfulness of those about him. The individual is sleepy during the daytime but sleepless at night. The pains of the Mercurius vivus patient are worse at night. The person's face is pale; the tongue and gums are swollen, teeth are loose, saliva is profuse, breath is foul; condition of the abdominal organs is sluggish; all the muscles are sore; and there is bone pain at night and in damp weather. In the most advanced state a generally heavy and soggy condition is found. The patient is inclined to be filthy in body, groveling mentally, and inclined to rambling incoherence or apathetic dementia.

Petroleum raffinatum (aka Benzinum petroleum)

I'm the king of the world

> Liking to be quicker than others
> As if everything is accelerating
> Head numbness like after hours of driving
> Alcohol craving
> Skeptical

Boredom

Sudden wakefulness/sudden fatigue

Psychological features of the remedy were illuminated by a proving conducted by master homeopath Sunil Anand in 1999 where the similarities with Fluoricum acidum were marked.

Power

- The oppressor who uses his power
- The victim of the power
- The global effects of the power game

The Oppressor

- Has a flamboyant lifestyle
- Exhibits peculiar personality traits
- Demonstrates a lawless survival mechanism

Several weeks into his presidency Donald Trump signed orders greasing the rails for the Keystone XL and Dakota Access oil pipelines. This action suggested yet another syphilitic remedy, Petroleum raffinatum, also called Benzinum petroleum (Benz-p). The ubiquity of petroleum is stunning. Its presence dominates transportation fuels; fuel oils for heating and electricity generation; asphalt and road oil; food stocks for making chemicals, plastics, and synthetic materials; pharmaceuticals; birth control devices; and, in other words, virtually every aspect of human existence. To learn how all of this came about, the 2015 James Corbett documentary, *How Big Oil Conquered the World,* is recommended. Also kindred in spirit is the 2007 Paul Thomas Anderson film, *There Will Be Blood.*

A syphilitic conundrum opposing entropy and consolidation forms the psychodrama playing out in petroleum's formation. As also applies to its precursor states, shale or kerogen, petroleum reflects a mortified consciousness pertaining to buried and compressed (consolidated) organic material that would have preferred participation in the life cycle within biodynamic soil (the perversion of which destiny is entropic).

Instead, like the mythic genie in the bottle, a great servant imprisoned in a jar is cast into the sea to brood over his lost utility, and a powerful but compressed rage builds and builds deep within the earth. Benzene, petroleum's refined product, eventually comes to vent this rage via its use in combustion and a vengeful, polluting havoc rained down upon its native soil birthplace.

Lifestyle Features

- Sybarite; needs enjoyment and stimulation. Uses or deals drugs, narcotics, and so on.
- Exploits appearance as a means of flaunting his authority. Clothes are flashy and trendy.
- Extravagance.
- Striking materialism. Must possess only the latest gadgets and a surplus of everything.

Personality Traits

- Highly competitive. Nothing less than the best can suffice. Being the first matters the most.
- Vengeful to contemporaries and potential rivals, with whom he is ruthless.
- Actions are quick so as to outstrip all the others. Drawn to racing cars, speedboats, and the like.
- Selfish.
- Can also procrastinate and postpone matters of concern to others.
- Flaunts his wealth or physical body for power and fame.

Survival Mechanisms

- At home with illegal transactions, black marketing, and similar questionable activities.
- Hoards money and other resources.
- Uses abusive language toward his inferiors.
- Exploits others; is willing to cheat and deceive.
- Takes refuge in violence, threats, conspiracies, assassination, entertainments.

Syphilinum

A wall between society and myself

Obsessive/compulsive	Circular thinking
Germophobic	Illicit sex/depravity
Stuck in foreplay	Secrecy/shame
Precocious	

Earlier in the chapter the syphilitic miasm was discussed. The miasm's nosode Syphilinum, made from a syphilitic discharge, is basically a mirror image of its pharmaceutical antagonist mercury. In clinical practice the two medicines are complementary.

Out Damned Spot!

Sexual activity, since it leads to reproduction and perpetuation of legacy, provides our hedge against entropy. But sexual activity can also be illicit, taking place secretly, in the dark, or in damp and nasty environs. The Syphilinum remedy reflects or promotes a dysfunctional hedge against entropy, a despairing sense of guilt, megalomania, and rage against contamination.

The Syphilinum remedy's mental symptoms include recursive logic and precocity, memory loss, and obsessive-compulsiveness pertaining to germ phobia. Isolation and struggle are expressed in suicidal ideas and antisocial behaviors. Physical symptoms include prostration and putrefying abscesses and ulcerations. Sexual addiction may be a prominent feature. In the miasmatic remedy state, an individual is caught up in a hopelessly circular desire for satisfaction akin to being stuck in sexual foreplay. Circular thinking digs a groove in the psyche. In its round and round perseveration the thinking groove deepens, engendering ever more severe alienation. A mental chasm separating the individual from society is thus carved.

Thulium

Fear of annihilation

Notions excessive and intemperate	Darkness, depths
Ultimate existential threat	Original sin
Wildness	Autoimmune disease
Sadomasochism	Alone

As of this writing, with the Russian invasion of Ukraine raging and the Doomsday Clock hovering at ninety seconds to midnight, the remedy Thulium merits a look, especially in regard to its fear-of-annihilation theme. Brought to light by Jan Scholten, Thulium is a late-stage remedy in the Lanthanide series; its theme concerns issues relating to autonomy (seeking, achieving, losing autonomy as a core problem). Individuals needing Thulium emanate seriousness and manifest symptoms involving heaviness. It is as if an enveloping darkness constrains their independence. In keeping with syphilitic guilt and shame, they are deluded that they are cursed by original sin or some other embedded evil. The individual is thus implicated in an onrushing annihilation. The radical disjunct is that a traumatized psyche buys into the argument, allowing the autonomy-infringing nihilism most feared to, in fact, manifest. Wildness, sadomasochism, and other dark and excessive behaviors erupt.

The delusion reflects or prompts autoimmune disease susceptibility. Additional pathologies that Scholten associates with Thulium include migraine headache, eye diseases, lung diseases (granulomas, pneumoconiosis, bronchitis, pneumonia, tuberculosis), liver problems (necrosis, fatty degeneration), spleen and kidney problems, numerous fertility problems for both men and women, arthritis, melanoma and vitiligo, blood coagulation and platelet issues, colitis, and diarrhea. It was noted earlier that the remedy Stramonium is also about fear of annihilation. Thulium, however, is absent Stramonium's trademark rage.

Comparison with Positronium

A remedy to compare with Thulium that also features fear or expectation of annihilation is Positronium, a remedy derived from an electron and its antiparticle, a positron, bound together into an unstable "exotic" atom. The positron's instability reflects the two particles' tendency to annihilate one another almost on contact. When this actually happens a pair of gamma ray photons is produced. Made up of both particle and antiparticle, Positronium represents a state midway between matter and antimatter. Its theme evinces impending cataclysm and the threat of annihilation. A Positronium remedy state features resignation, weakness, and a sinking sensation. Its terrain encompasses the heart and blood circulation, the nervous system, and the immune system. Positive features of someone needing this remedy include intellectual curiosity and an affinity for the structure of things.

In addition to treatment within TCM, homeopathy, and biomedicine, a number of therapeutic practices may promote health within the sense dimension of Hearing.

Hearing Dimension Health Promotion Practices
- Be moderate in all things.
- Secure your family's safety and security.
- Improve your community.
- Nurture the mother of Hearing, Smell: Strive to remain centered.
- Maintain good body heat.
- Find and fulfill your life's meaning and mission.
- Consider and secure your legacy.

5

Will the insurrection of my birth prove fruitful?

Cancer Miasm • Sight • Wood Phase •
Anger • Liver–Gall Bladder

The world was getting along perfectly well until you came around. Your arrival on earth was thus an insurrection versus the status quo. The question is, will your existence leave a lasting impression or pass by scarcely noticed? As the words emblazoned on his memorial statue in Washington, DC, *Non inutilis vixi* (I have not lived in vain), indicate, the question mattered to Samuel Hahnemann, father of homeopathy, who led a momentous insurrection against the forces of conventional medicine.

THE CANCER MIASM AND
THE SENSE DIMENSION OF SIGHT

Does my self-worth depend on perfectionism or self-sacrifice? Have I mounted a successful rebellion against my family of birth? Do I have a vision for the future? In a chaotic world, do I wield my hammer of anger creatively? The trio Peter, Paul, and Mary set the example in 1963 with their song "If I Had a Hammer," singing, "I'd hammer out danger, I'd hammer out a warning, I'd hammer out love between my brothers and my sisters, all over this land." Such questions at the

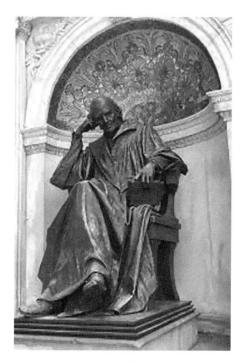

Non inutilis vixi
Samuel Hahnemann memorial, Washington, DC

core of the sense dimension of Sight underlie pathology within the cancer miasm.

The Sense Dimension of Sight

Wuxing phase: Wood
Emotion: Anger
Organ: Liver–Gall Bladder
Theme: Creativity vs. chaos

Sight and insight are inextricably combined. To see the light, to see the truth, sets us free. But vision is panoramic. By taking in everything, like Adam and Eve we perceive too much and absorb more knowledge than can be handled. Seeing with new eyes that they were naked prompted Adam and Eve to experience an unfamiliar and puzzling emotion: shame. Sightlessness, however, offers scant solace as it can open the door to chaos, in which case better not to emulate King Lear and acquire insight at the price of going blind.

Sight interprets the chaos of light, converting it into brilliant, creative, and meaningful images. Through sight we are active rather than passive viewers of a completed world of objects. Meeting the world and constructing interpretations that take light into account via sight, our vision is fundamentally creative. It imposes order and pattern on the chaos of photons. If we fail to compose relevant images from the irritating maze and ambiguity of visual stimuli, we fall prey to predators and the hazards of potholes or onrushing traffic. Every shift in our visual field calls us to react and to creatively transform irritating visual stimuli into meaningful images.

Ungrounded creativity (delusion, fantasy, hallucination) is an invitation to chaos. But on the other hand, when our vision is insufficiently creative, constraints and galling limitations dim the light beckoning us to liberty. The appropriate emotional reaction to constraint, even that which is self-imposed, is anger. Turned inward upon the self, anger can manifest as depression. When anger is consuming, insight is lost. When blind with rage, the possibility of creative response is forfeit. Anger's resolution involves recovery of unseen possibilities, re-envisioning a situation, seeing matters in a new light. The distinction between chaos and anger is a matter of choice.

No one is ever truly and completely blind. Blindsight, the ability to perceive elements of the environment even when the brain's visual lobes do not function, was confirmed in 2008 in a report by a team of international researchers of a patient with bilateral damage to the primary visual (striate) cortex who navigated around numerous barriers placed along a long corridor.[1] The ability to see nonvisually reflects the firing of neurons located deep in the midbrain, where subconscious activation promotes intuition-like awareness. Because not only the eye but also the entire body appears to respond visually, healthy vision is confirmed to involve the creative interpretation of photons. We are never truly, entirely blind.

WOOD PHASE AND
TRADITIONAL CHINESE MEDICINE

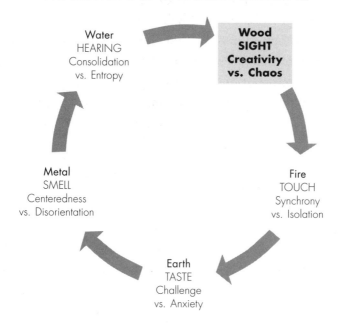

Water
HEARING
Consolidation
vs. Entropy

Wood
SIGHT
Creativity
vs. Chaos

Metal
SMELL
Centeredness
vs. Disorientation

Fire
TOUCH
Synchrony
vs. Isolation

Earth
TASTE
Challenge
vs. Anxiety

Because Wood within Wuxing pertains to the spring, this phase exemplifies the energy of growth, change, and pushing through obstacles. It is a very active energy and denotes a spirit of decisive action and rebirth. What does this have to do with the cancer miasm? Spirited action does not occur with decisive choice. The issue of free choice looms large within this miasm, as we shall see.

Carcinosinum across
the Miasmatic Spectrum

We learned earlier that the tubercular miasm is comorbid with both sycosis and the syphilitic miasm. Now we find that the cancer miasm is comorbid with the other four miasms: tuberculinum, psora, sycosis, and syphilis. Another way to explain this is through the materia medica of the cancer nosode (in this case, tissue from breast carcinoma), Carcinosinum. The Carcinosinum remedy expresses themes from all previous miasms and, not surprisingly, from all five of the sense dimensions as well.

In the Sense Dimension of Touch

The core issue is the tension between synchrony and isolation. Normal cells unselfishly serve the synchrony of a greater good related to the needs of the surrounding community of tissue. With corruption into a cancer cell, the cell degrades into isolation. Consequently, at cellular and psychological levels, the core tension between isolation and synchrony is increased. The Carcinosinum remedy state depicts an experience of preternatural responsibility at an early age, leading to an excessively sympathetic adult. The isolated cancer cell and the isolation a cancer patient are related: A child compelled to be a caretaker for an adult creates both a martyr-like delusion that her own needs must be sacrificed for those of others and isolation, an enduring sense that she must carry the burden alone.

In the Sense Dimension of Taste

A rapidly growing tumor's aggressive and hedonistic appropriation of resources may be considered bacterial consciousness run amok. This mirrors a wild exaggeration of Taste's hunger for challenge, the positive pole in the challenge versus anxiety dichotomy. Someone mired in the Carcinosinum remedy state manifests a version of this excess, being as maniacal and workaholic as a tumor cell. On the anxiety pole, an individual evinces perfectionism and fastidiousness.

In the Sense Dimension of Smell

The metastatic inclination of cancer cells to travel expresses as the desire to travel; not being content with where one is reflects being uncentered, the negative pole of the sense dimension of Smell's centeredness-versus-disorientation dichotomy. So does its romantic affinity for distant locales, far afield from its place of origin. On the physical plane Carcinosinum is prescribed for asthma, bronchitis, café-au-lait pigmentation and numerous moles, and lung and skin conditions that pertain to Smell.

As previously discussed, disorientation operating at the genetic level is implicated in frameshift mutation–related Smell-dimension cancers of the breast and large intestine.

In the Sense Dimension of Hearing

A perverse expression of consolidation is expressed in genetic predisposition to one or more cancers. Genetically, a heritable mutation of a gene on the thirteenth human chromosome creates a susceptibility to the deactivation of a tumor suppressor, which, in turn, allows tumors to grow in the retina and other locales. Thus, familial retinoblastoma arises due to its having been imprinted upon and consolidated within Kidney yang. Carcinosinum, the principal remedy relevant to the cancer miasm, is at play, applicable to cancers imprinted and consolidated within the germ line.

In the Sense Dimension of Sight

Cancer cells exhibit a perverse creativity in forming novel mutant combinations. Here tumor growth is an exaggeration of the negative pole of chaos, demonstrated by the juxtaposition of incompatible tissues. Pertaining to Sight, symptoms related to Carcinosinum include twitching of the eyes or limbs, emotional sensitivity, and a will to be productive.

It is the Carcinosinum mindset that tells the full story. Every birth is an insurrection against the status quo. The world ran perfectly well until you came along. But for your insurrection to be fruitful over the course of a lifetime, a successful rebellion (particularly against parents) must be mounted in order that you become a fully independent human being. Someone needing Carcinosinum, having failed to mount a successful rebellion, struggles thereafter to differentiate himself.

Recapitulating sense dimensional themes, we have the myth of Scylla. In the *Odyssey,* the magnificent ancient Greek epic by Homer, Ulysses was sailing home to his wife Penelope when his ship confronted the narrow Strait of Messina guarded by two terrifying monsters, Scylla and Charybdis, entrenched on either side of the strait. According to the myth, the beautiful nymph Scylla had been poisoned in her bath and transformed into a hideous monster with twelve feet and six heads, each with three rows of teeth. Below the waist her body was composed of monstrous dogs that barked unceasingly. In this state she was destined to live forever in unending misery and loathing (Touch), rooted in her spot and eviscerating all within her reach.

> *Before the gates there sat*
> *On either side a formidable Shape.*
> *The one seemed a woman to the waist, and fair,*
> *But ended foul in many a scaly fold,*
> *Voluminous and vast—a serpent armed*
> *With mortal sting. About her middle round*
> *A cry of Hell-hounds never-ceasing barked*
> *With wide Cerberean mouths full loud, and rung*
> *A hideous peal; yet, when they list, would creep,*
> *If aught disturbed their noise, into her womb,*
> *And kennel there; yet there still barked and howled*
> *Within unseen. Far less abhorred than these*
> *Vexed Scylla, bathing in the sea that parts*
> *Calabria from the hoarse Trinacrian shore.*
>
> JOHN MILTON,
> *PARADISE LOST,* BOOK II

Just as Scylla was transformed by poison (Hearing) into a gruesome monster, so once innocent cells may become malignant through damage from macrocosmic and microcosmic exposures. Scylla's voraciousness reflects the relentlessly invasive and devouring hunger of cancer. To the extent that there are no limits on how many times cancer cells are able to divide, they share another of Scylla's traits—immortality. Similarly, Scylla's isolation (Touch) and self-loathing (Smell) are manifested in cancer cells. To use biologist Robert Weinberg's term, a "renegade" cancer cell alienates itself from its own community (Sight), thereby instigating a bodily outcry and a self-directed witch hunt. Scylla's chaotic anatomy (Sight) correlates with cancer's breakdown of normal order and the chaotic management of cell replacement. Tumors known as *teratomata*

(Greek: monster tumor) consist of tissues well enough differentiated to contain hair and teeth (Hearing) that may be either malignant or benign. Echoes from multiple levels of consciousness and experience are retained in the myth of Scylla, herself a teratomata sprung to life.

CREATIVITY VERSUS CHAOS

We now discuss how creativity and chaos are opposed.

Creativity

Optimally engaged, the sense dimension of Sight is decisive, discerning, and liberating. Consistent with the Liver's role in the promotion of flow, the creative aspect of Sight bypasses the ego and the will so as to manifest according to John Keats's expression, "Beauty is truth, truth beauty." Keats is saying that creative action at its best is purity of vision, an all-encompassing awareness of possibility.

We ought not assume that sensitivities are entirely inborn. Sensitivity to the nuances of music, the story told by a painting, and the suffering of others can be cultivated. Unless the capability to influence sensitivity exists, inner knowledge has little value with regard to health. Susceptibility to illness, too, is rooted within the tenor of our thoughts and choices. Mental hygiene matters because whether our dreams are nightmares or visions of glory, they will manifest in our day-to-day lives. Independent of treatment, an individual's sensitivity and his ability to heal are inseparable. A shift in sensitivity, whether for better or for worse, has diagnostic import for a homeopath.

Chaos

In Greek mythology Khaos, or Chaos, was conceived to be the first of the primeval gods and to represent the void of infinite space from which everything in creation is birthed. According to the Roman poet Ovid, circa year 8 CE, Chaos was a confused mass containing the elements of all created things.

Chaos personified the abyss or unformed matter, the opposite of birth and creativity on the creativity/chaos axis, the core issue in the

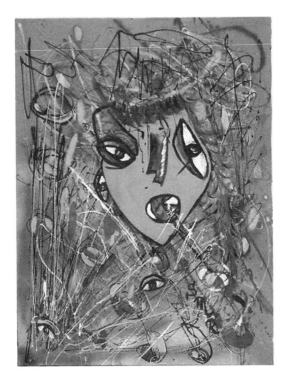

La Rage, oil painting by Siminiuc Mouline Radia; anger transformed into creativity

dimension of Sight. Chaos manifests through indecision, delusion, anger, or through being visually, cognitively, or spiritually overwhelmed. When chaos erupts, outrage is prompted. It is best then to respond with inspiration and creativity.

These traits of chaos are major gateways to the stagnation of Liver chi and they imply the existence of different disorders and different remedy states. Neurological chaos within Traditional Chinese Medicine also comes under the Liver's umbrella. Though the concept of nerves and a nervous system is lacking, an equivalent exists within Liver functionality. The Liver is said to govern the body's tendons, whose ability to contract and release was held to include what Western science refers to as neurological function. Symptoms such as ticks, twitches, cramps, and seizures, because they appear and move randomly throughout the body, seemed wind-like to the ancient Chinese. The chaotic nature of these symptoms earned them the sobriquet of Liver wind.

The Cancer Miasm's Existential Themes

- Am I free or am I a follower?
- Does my self-worth reflect only what I can do for others?
- How do I counter the chaos of the world?
- At what cost a successful rebellion?
- Is there a vision for the future?
- Is my life meaningful?

TREATMENTS AND EXPECTATIONS

Remedies manifesting subcategories of *Will the insurrection of my birth prove fruitful?*

Cadmium metallicum	Stramonium
Carcinosinum	Veratrum album
Cicuta virosa	Yersinia pestis
Plumbum metallicum	

Cadmium metallicum

Creativity's last gasp

Indifference	Must discharge (better: eruption)
Exaggerated creativity	Violent insanity
Cancer	Decay

The tension between creativity and chaos and the need to sustain creative vision finds expression in the remedy Cadmium metallicum. Individuals needing this remedy are despondent and apathetic and have a loathing of life. They cannot concentrate, say and do the wrong things, or misplace items, such as putting their cell phones in the refrigerator. Their dreams are vivid, anxious, or about sickness, leaving them full of worry upon awakening. They can avoid people and be averse to music and noise. Odors and disagreeable notions make them nauseous. Violent transitions from impulsivity to irritability and deep depression create an impression of insanity.

Physical symptoms of the remedy state include vertigo; visual field problems, such as objects appearing to recede and return; neuralgic headaches, maddening pressing pains throughout whole head extending to eyes and ears; mushy stool, constipation. and intestinal pain; joint pain; and numbness of feet and hands while sitting. When the profile fits, Cadmium is an important remedy in the treatment of cancer.

Jan Scholten's analysis of the remedy is that its late-stage position (stage 12) in the periodic table's silver row, pertaining to creativity, provides the theme: Decay and repetition in the performance of the arts. Thus, as compensation for having run out of ideas, the individual is prone to exaggeration in creating art.

Avatars of Cadmium are Salvador Dali and Vincent van Gogh. If an artist's work is far ahead of its time the artist may feel powerless for much the same reason and fall into a Cadmium state. To cover up his sense of powerlessness he can become stubborn or arrogant. The art will tend to become repetitive, to have an artificial quality, or to parody itself. A need to bolster loss of power may draw him to forgery. Also, an academic pressured to annually publish or perish may be drawn into Cadmium after his best ideas have already been perfectly expressed. In this sense, and as I have seen in my clinical experience with the remedy, the Cadmium metallicum person was initially innovative for the time and punished for that. Their extreme positions and emotions make them enemies in the arts or in their particular areas of expertise.

Carcinosinum

A false freedom

Incomplete rebellion	Overadaptation to others' needs
Love of travel/metastasis	Romance/love of nature
Cancer/cell seduced by a lie	Neurological ticks

Though Carcinosinum is represented across all the miasms, being a nosode made from carcinoma its primary affinity is with the cancer misam. Individuals needing it have a coffee-colored complexion and, usually, numerous dark moles on the skin. They crave spicy foods, butter, and chocolate. They have a tendency to become constipated and experience twitchiness of the limbs and sometimes of the face. The remedy state reflects or promotes susceptibility to cancer. The twitchings pertain to the sense dimension of Sight's dominion over neurological function.

Reflecting the Consciousness of the Cancer Cell

Cancer cells have been seduced into accepting an illusion: that their loyalty belongs not to the organism at large but to a family of tumor cells, membership of which grants them immortality. Unlike humble, mortal, non-cancer cells, cancer cells can replicate endlessly. Awareness that the tumor eventually kills its host, terminating the cancer cell as well, is denied. In parallel fashion the psyche of a Carcinosinum individual is subliminally invested in everlasting life. This is evident from an excess of sympathy that is both debilitating and self-destructive. One of my patients had obsessive concern for her ancient and terminally ill pet that allowed her to spare no expense in preventing its death. Another patient, unable to consent to a stoppage of life support under any circumstance, rejected a loved one's request that he be her health care proxy.

At the mind-body level, susceptibility to the tumor's argument lies in the individual's insecurity and failure to mount an individuating and developmentally important rebellion early in life. In turn this susceptibility may have been fed by having been burdened with an excess of familial responsibilty when a child. In consequence the individual has become overadapted to the needs of others, incapable of saying no.

To extend the parallel, cancer cells are ambitious, hardworking, and willing to engage in self-sacrificing behavior. In metastasis, cancer cells reveal themselves to be romantics willing to travel to distant locales, where they eagerly colonize tissue whose nature is entirely foreign to the tissue of their origin. Carcinosinum individuals, who relish travel to distant lands, have no compunction about carrying full responsibility for any task they accept.

As Within, So Without:
John Milton's Image of Satan

By externalizing and objectifying our fears, myths like that of Scylla alleviate our helplessness. The myth of Satan does us the same service. In many world religions Satan is a fallen angel, formerly favored by God. The myth of Satan is viewed allegorically as the cultural and biological equivalent of cancer willfully seeking freedom from, and chaotically ruling, our bodies. Like Satan, cancer engineers the creation of a self-immolating hell. We return once more to John Milton's epic poem, *Paradise Lost,* where in dramatic fashion Satan's power to seduce through overpowering charisma is on display. Not for nothing is he notorious as the "Father of Lies."

> Hail, horrors! Hail, infernal world! and thou, profoundest Hell, Receive thy new possessor—one who brings a mind not to be changed by place or time. The mind is its own place, and in itself can make a heaven of hell, a hell of heaven. What matter where, if I be still the same, and what I should be, all but less than he whom thunder hath made greater? Here at least we shall be free.
>
> JOHN MILTON, *PARADISE LOST,* BOOK I

Cicuta virosa
Retreat into childhood

Head trauma	Estranged from society
Palsy	Want of trust
Grimacing	Childish

Made from water hemlock, the neurological medicine Cicuta virosa features the radical disjunct "excessive reactivity fosters dullness." A distortion of perspective and a sense that objects are either too close or too distant speaks to an overall balance in the remedy picture.

The Cicuta virosa individual is excessively naïve. The remedy reflects or promotes this individual thinking and behaving like a child. As we see in sensitive children, there is a heightened reactivity. There is distrustfulness and a sense of being estranged from society. When the feelings of such a person, child or adult, are deeply hurt, the reaction is systemic and severe. Convulsiveness and the chaos of neurological overactivity is prompted. Vision symptoms are numerous. We find a tendency to stare blankly and also diplopia (double vision). When reading, letters disappear or travel up and down; objects approach and recede or appear black; figures in the visual field vacillate. Vision in sunlight is poor or random, and momentary loss of vision occurs.

Along with Cocculus indicus, Cicuta virosa is a major remedy for convulsions resulting from fright or an injury to the brain. It is also prominent in the treatment of grand mal seizure—also known as tonic-clonic seizure—with a loss of consciousness and violent muscle contractions.

Plumbum metallicum

Sic semper tyrannus

Neurological deadening	Assassination (always to tyrants)
Sense of order	Toppled from a high place
Reductionistic reasoning	Visual snow
Heavy sensation/robotic	Sudden blindness/convulsion
Nonreactive/constipation	Violent thoughts

At the mental/emotional level the Plumbum metallicum state's famous keynote fear is of being assassinated. Assassination is the punishment one might expect for one who occupies a position of great authority and power, such as a king or dictator. For this reason the Plumbum metallicum individual can be an organized, controlling, high-level performer. As one of the perquisites of a person in an elevated position is an extravagant lifestyle, you may see Plumbum come up for someone who has indulged himself in food, drink, and sex. Not surprisingly, Plumbum is prominent in rubrics pertaining to feeling alone and destructiveness, as well as violent thoughts and a suicidal disposition.

Made from a profound neurological toxin—lead—the remedy Plumbum also comes into play for diminished intelligence due to lead poisoning and for wooden, robotic movement. The remedy addresses generally sclerotic conditions. Its domain is the muscles, nerves, spinal cord, abdomen, kidneys, blood vessels, and blood. Onset of Plumbum conditions is gradual, insidious, and progressive, though violent changeability of character and incoherent speech will suddenly surface. In keeping with the sense dimension of Sight, Plumbum metallicum is a prominent resource in the event of sudden blindness.

Visual snow syndrome involves the visual field being saturated with flickering dots of static. According to the American Academy of Ophthalmology (AAO), it is "a form of visual hallucination characterized by the perception of small, bilateral, simultaneous, diffuse, mobile, asynchronous dots usually throughout the entire visual field . . . present in all conditions of illumination, even with the eyes closed."[2] Its neurology is akin to that of migraine headache. The AAO adds that patients experiencing visual snow appear to have both cortical hyperexcitability and loss of inhibition of visual processing in the thalamo-cortico circuitry within the primary visual cortex. The thalamus is the body's information relay station. Apart from smell, all sensory inputs are processed within the brain's thalamus before being sent to the cerebral cortex for interpretation. Irregular function in the thalamus disrupts sleep and wakeful consciousness.

The trajectory of the state toward paralysis can feature hysterical and infantile behavior. The muscles can be flaccid and emaciated; as with wrist drop, the joints can suddenly be dysfunctional; a strong polarity involves hyperaesthesia (hypersensitivity of the skin) that is worse from touch and convulsive trembling and jerking of the limbs. Muscular and violent contraction is prominent as in retraction—of abdomen, anus, testes, navel. There are lightning pains. Plumbum is a major remedy for chronic epilepsy with marked aura, cramps, multiple sclerosis, spinal sclerosis, anemia, jaundice, arteriosclerosis, and hypertension.

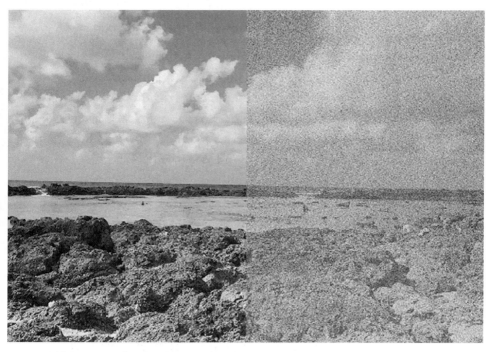

Illustration of typical vision at left, contrasted with example of visual
snow syndrome in the optic field at right

Photo by Kara Perricone on AllAboutVision.com

Stramonium

Abandoned in the wilderness

PTSD from terror and violence	Painlessness
Violent rage	Convulsion
Beseeching/raving/devout	Affected by glitter, bright light

We encountered this remedy earlier when, in the context of the Inborn
Toolkit, Stramonium was referenced as embodying excessive use of the
hammer of anger. Presently we reference it as exemplifying inability to
convert anger into creativity. This remedy, made from the thorn apple
plant (jimsonweed) or the related plant datura, must always be considered for PTSD victims, such as war veterans returning to society.
Individuals needing Stramonium have experienced abandonment or
witnessed terror so severe as to project them into a netherland located

somewhere betwixt life and death. They feel like a child completely abandoned in the wilderness. Their body can seem so unalive as to feel woodenly impervious to pain, and bodily functions can become stifled.

At the opposite pole even the most minimal threat is for such a person a crisis of survival, offering no option other than to dredge from the inner depths a desperate and primal response. This is the remedy's keynote feature: explosive rage, raving mania, or frantic prayer. Sensitivity to glittering or glimmering light is found, presumably reflecting off the weapon he glimpsed, representing both the terror and hope lurking within the darkness of abandonment. A Stramonium individual is also prone to beseeching requests and religious frenzy. On the physical level there is trembling of the whole body, especially of the lips, hands, and feet; violent jerking in the arms; and lameness of the legs. The tongue hangs out of the mouth. The individual is prone to murmuring and displays loss of reason.

Dimension of Sight symptoms include staring eyes, dilated pupils, loss of vision, complaints that all is dark, and calling out for light. Or small objects look large, or all objects look black. Other symptoms include night blindness, green vision, objects appearing crooked or jumbled, and the onset of total blindness.

Veratrum album

So lost, only I know the way

Loss of social position	Self-righteous
Collapse from fear	Egotism
Precocity/mania	Stomach cold/anguish

In this remedy made from white hellebore we find the effects of being gripped by the pliers of fear, desperation to reconcile creativity with chaos, and a multileveled distortion of vision. Veratrum album is indicated for one who due to having had the rug pulled out from under him has experienced loss of social position. The trauma may have involved the unwelcome intrusion into his family of a new and appealing sibling. Or an abusive stepparent has suddenly supplanted his loving father.

His experience is akin to eviction from Paradise. As *veratrum* means truth, the Veratrum album person dons the self-righteous and boastful camouflage of being the sole bearer of truth. The radical disjunct can be framed: *I am so lost, only I know the way.* This can fit the passionate leader of a cult, a frenzied religious apostle, or an overly zealous preacher. Associated symptoms include sudden exhaustion, nausea, a state of collapse, and numerous mental derangements. A visual delusion that his portion of food is invariably smaller than that of a dining companion as well as many forms of hysteria can also be found. On a positive note, the remedy state reflects but also promotes precocity.

A Veratrum album Avatar, Aron Nimzowitsch

Well-known in the world of chess is Aron Nimzowitsch, whose personality and misadventures vividly depict Veratrum album's key features. This nineteenth-century chess prodigy wrote a hugely ambitious text on chess theory that uniquely and cogently presents the game's principles. His book, *My System,* was not fully appreciated in his lifetime. Justifying his hypermodern concepts exasperated Nimzowitsch, especially when he lost tournament games. Unable to fully manifest his brilliant theories made him defensive and self-righteous. When dining out Nimzowitsch was notorious for being certain his portion was always the smallest. Following defeat by an inferior player he would scream, "Why must I lose to this idiot?" Where smoking was banned in tournament halls his opponents unnerved the volatile Nimzowitsch by placing unlit cigars next to their chess pieces, exploiting his investment in a chess precept that the threat is stronger than its execution.

The traumatized Veratrum album person carries with him an expectation of the rug being yanked or of approval being withheld. His fear provokes reenactment of the drama in physical terms, as in sudden collapse of energy and sudden nausea. On the mental and emotional plane, frenzy, distractibility, clinginess, hypersensitivity, touchiness, and vigilance are evident. The remedy's domain is the mind, nerves, abdomen, heart, blood, blood vessels, respiration, vertex (top of head), and digestive system. The state features copious evacuations such as vomiting, purging, salivating, sweating, and urinating. There is profound prostration, coldness, blueness of the skin, sudden sinking of energy, cold perspiration on the forehead with all complaints, and frequent ice-cold chill.

Yersinia pestis
The horror of the world

Global horror (bubonic plague)

Sabotage of authority

Inverted idealism

Thwarted cathartic anger (hammer of anger suppressed)

Shadowy existence

Too smart for your own good

Stomach ailments/ulcer

We conclude our discussion of existential remedies with a medicine whose theme matches the most common denotation of an existential problem. In connection with the crisis of unavoidable climate change or the likelihood of nuclear war, for example: "Oh God! We're all going to die!" Yersinia pestis, made from the bubonic plague bacterium, concerns awareness of a horror afflicting the world. Those in touch with or dealing with its inner workings manifest thwarted and loosened rage as well as major distortions of perspective.

An infection of the lymphatic system, the bubonic plague usually results from the bite of an infected flea, the type often found on rodents, such as rats. After the rodent host dies the fleas seek other hosts within whom the lymph nodes become embattled. In a vulnerable individual *Yersinia pestis* resists phagocytosis, the cellular process for eliminating microorganisms, foreign substances, and damaged cells.

In the disease's progression the lymph nodes hemorrhage and become necrotic. Though "bubonic plague" is often used synonymously with "plague," it refers specifically to an infection that enters through the skin and without treatment kills about 50 percent of infected patients in four to seven days. The bubonic plague is believed by many to be the Black Death that swept through Europe in the 1340s.

Louis Klein can be thanked for bringing forth the essence of this remedy whose theme reflects a deep level of self-sabotage. He describes the personalty of the Yersinia pestis person as someone friendly to the point of being supplicating and idealizing of another (such as one in the role of knowledgeable professional). But then in a quick turn of events the individual flips and seeks to destroy you. Such individuals have been accurately diagnosed as having borderline personalities and are candidates for fringe positions in society. My belief is that their treacherous dynamic reenacts a prior trauma in which they were punished for harboring idealistic aspirations. As in Stockholm syndrome, the Yersinia pestis individual appears to adopt the vile means of retribution that was suffered.[3]

What might be the connection between this mindset, rats, and the bubonic plague? The answer may be embedded in the famous fable "The Pied Piper of Hamelin," a legend from the Middle Ages. A pipe-playing ratcatcher dressed in multicolored clothing was hired by the town to lure rats away with his magic pipe. Ungrateful citizens refused to pay for this promised service and so he retaliated by using his instrument's magical power on their children, leading them away as he had the rats. This version of the story spread as folklore and has appeared in the writings of Johan Wolfgang von Goethe, the Brothers Grimm, Robert Browning, and others.

We saw in my interpretation of the tuberculosis miasm that those willing to countenance rampant human squalor, congestion, and filth are at fault. Rat symbolism appearing throughout history in myths, culture, and the arts indicates such animals have a taboo status due to their presence in unhygienic conditions, thuggery, gangsterism, and shadowy power plays. Normally found in the sewers, they represent the lower strata of society as well as cruelty, poverty, sadism, and eroticism. If the bubonic plague is teaching a similar moral lesson, the Pied Piper fable pertains. Could it concern the unjustified belief that the goodness of existence can be taken for granted, its bounty limitlessly available for plunder?

✧ ✧ ✧

Failure to bypass chaos so that vital creative options can be perceived sets the energetic stage for a number of chronic illnesses. A decades-long process of minor decrements and compromises in thought, deed, and vision may be entailed, but as the accretion of ills tends to be imperceptible, maintenance of good hygiene within Sight is recommended. Several therapeutic practices can help promote health within the sense dimension of Sight.

Sight Dimension Health Promotion Practices

- Clearly, cleanly attend to detail.
- Convert anger into creative action.
- Nurture health in the other sense dimensions.
- See the big picture.
- Foster flow in all situations.
- Adopt simplicity; avoid clutter.
- Think like a world citizen.

In the Strait of Messina

*Navigating between the Scylla of Cancer
and the Charybdis of Chronic Illness*

The existential challenge of thriving into old age involves a challenging feat. Like Ulysses at the end of his long homeward voyage, we must navigate between two hazards, the Scylla of cancer on the one side and the Charybdis of chronic illness on the other. In the *Odyssey*, as Ulysses's ship passed through the narrow Strait of Messina, the enormous tidal whirlpool of the sea monster-goddess Charybdis swirled on one side of the strait opposite the equally dangerous monster Scylla, whom we have seen is the perfect embodiment of cancer. In one ancient story describing the origin of Charybdis, she was a daughter of the divine sea god Pontos and the earth goddess Gaia. Charybdis had so angered Zeus that he turned her into a monster compelled forever to suck water in and expel it out three times a day, drawing men down into the spiral whirlpool to their deaths. Charybdis symbolizes the cyclical, vortex nature of chronic illness.

The whirlpool-like dynamic governing Wuxing's Five Phases serves to model both healthful function and pathology. It is a metaphysical scheme of classification in which TCM's organs and symptoms are assigned to particular phases. The term *phase* describes both the five core organizing categories and related processes occurring in the body throughout various stages of disease and healing. The primary phase is the generating (also called the *sheng*, nourishing, or promotion) cycle. Deviations from the healthful movement of the generating cycle—disharmonized energetic relationship within the system—include the *ko*

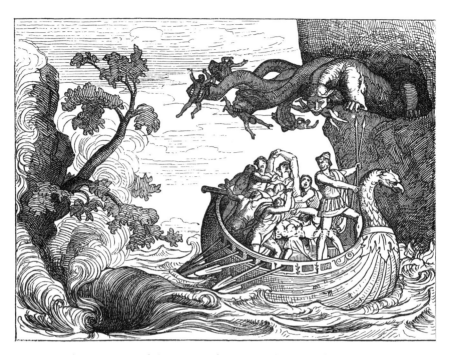

Steel engraving of the Strait of Messina by A. H. Payne, 1840

(regulating or control) cycle, destructive (*cheng* or overacting sequence) cycle, and anti-ko (*wu* or insulting sequence) cycle. Sense dimensional analysis appropriates these dynamics in order to provide a template upon which conventional (biomedical) illness and existential quandaries can be superimposed.

WUXING'S RELATED PHASES THROUGH DISEASE AND HEALING

Wuxing's phases describe the energy transformation from one state to another. Think of them as metaphysical (or energetic) agents of change.

Smooth Sailing, the Generating Cycle

In the first of these, the generating cycle, each phase is viewed as a mother, responsible for nurturing the growth and development of a succeeding (following) child phase. The mother supplies a generating force or foundation for the immediately following phase. The Fire phase provides a foundation for the Earth phase, the Earth element provides a nurturing foundation for the Metal phase, and so on. Pathologies may arise in these relationships, as when a particular mother phase fails to nourish her child phase, or a child phase drains energy from its mother. Clockwise movement through the phases traditionally models a beneficial flow of energy that we associate with developmental health.

The Controlling Cycle

The second main cycle, the controlling cycle, is involved in a checks-and-balances relationship that helps keep things in order. Each phase both controls and is controlled by another phase (for example, Water controls Fire but is itself controlled by Earth).

The Overcontrolling Cycle

The third main cycle, the overcontrolling cycle, is an exaggeration of the second cycle to a degree where pathology begins. Water, for example, can overdo its job of controlling Fire to the point of causing flooding (accounting for the symptom menorrhagia, for example).

The Insult Cycle

The fourth main cycle, the insult cycle, is suggestive of vengefulness or spite: A controlled phase rebels against its controlling master phase. High fever, for example, can be modeled as raging Fire counteracting against Water. Within TCM theory the resulting dehydration is termed yin depletion.

CONUNDRUM RESOLUTION

In ancient China, a Five Phases account of the physiological relationships holding between the five principal viscera sufficiently explained how the body worked. Over the years TCM theory grew more complex and the five viscera's interactions more intricate. Nevertheless, the Five Phases are useful for schematizing how resolution of a core conundrum promotes health whereas incomplete resolution lends itself to illness susceptibility. Serial resolution of dimensional themes defines the generating cycle and denotes health.

Heart Energy (Synchrony)
Promotes the Energy of the Spleen (Challenge)

Resolving isolation versus synchrony—relating to heart ailments, depression, schizophrenia, and autism—expresses mastery of Touch. The Heart being the source of synchrony, it generates not only the impetus of the blood, meaning its ability to circulate, but also that of the chi (the power underlying all functionality). Its energy promotes that of the Spleen, the organ embedded within the succeeding Earth phase. The Spleen's housing a desire for challenge so as to convert nutrients into blood that fuels the body's development describes the Spleen's domain over metabolism. This can be thought of as Fire creates ash, connoting Earth.

Spleen Energy (Challenge)
Promotes the Energy of the Lungs (Centeredness)

Resolving anxiety versus challenge—relating to gastrointestinal ailments, arthritis, diabetes, and anxiety—expresses mastery of Taste. In addition to providing nutrients for the growth and development of chi and blood, the Spleen holds responsibility for transporting, distributing, and transforming nutrients and for promoting fluid metabolism. The Lungs oversee respiration and also control the chi of the entire body, thereby assuring proper orientation to the external environment. In ensuring that its upward transportation of food essence nourishes the Lungs, the Spleen promotes its ability to perform respiration and disperse chi. (Mnemonic device: Metal is found in the Earth.)

Lung Energy (Centeredness)
Promotes the Energy of the Kidneys (Consolidation)

Resolving disorientation versus centeredness—relating to respiratory ailments, allergies, eczema, Alzheimer's, and grief—expresses mastery of Smell. The Lungs activate the flow of vital energy, blood, and body fluid. They also filter inspired air, directing it downward so that food essence in the upper body cavity is distributed throughout the body. This function also includes promotion of a principal function of the Kidneys. Fluid products of metabolism are directed downward into the Kidneys and the Urinary Bladder, where further filtration into turbid (subject to excretion) or clean (returned into circulation) fluid takes place.

In keeping with consolidation, the idea of converting the temporal into the permanent, the Kidneys latch on to the inspired breath and pull it into the lower *tan tien* (energy center), or cinnabar field. For the duration of time it can be held there, a touch of immortality is experienced. In many meditation (or centering) practices, respiration is radically slowed even to the point of coming to a complete standstill. Few can master this trance state during which respiration is unnecessary, known as samadhi. The rest of us are condemned to expire (in both senses of the word), relinquishing our hold of our indrawn breath and, in so doing, relinquishing our brief connection to the cinnabar field. (Mnemonic device: Metal can be melted down into a liquid form, Water.)

Kidney Energy (Consolidation)
Promotes the Energy of the Liver (Creativity)

Resolving entropy versus consolidation—relating to genitourinary ailments, bone loss, back pain, and epigenetic disorders—expresses mastery of Hearing. In physiological terms the Kidneys maintain the integrity of Water within the body. Kidney promotion of the Liver consists of holding responsibility for the bones, within which blood is created, and Water forms the material basis for blood, which is stored and released under the aegis of the Liver. The Kidneys house our inheritable energy. This consists of not only essence-related functions pertaining to growth and development but also talents and illness susceptibilities that have consolidated within our lineage. Thus, in the sense that our inherent talents and predispositions play a determining role with regard to the expression of our personal creativity, Kidney energy promotes that of the Liver. Creativity is strong when it has access to the unconscious, where our consolidated talents and predispositions repose. (Mnenomic device: Water promotes the growth of plants, Wood.)

Liver Energy (Creativity)
Promotes the Energy of the Heart (Synchrony)

Resolving chaos versus creativity—relating to neurological ailments, migraine, dysmenorrhea, and PTSD—expresses mastery of Sight. Although TCM does not consider that menstrual blood and circulatory blood are one and the same, when the Liver's management of blood movement is healthful, then the Heart has sufficiency of blood. For example, irresolvable disappointment and resentment produce a state of stagnation disruptive to metabolism and menstrual function in women. A resulting mineral imbalance disturbs the *shen,* the spirit housed within the Heart, as well as blood circulation. This accounts for such symptoms as dizziness, insomnia, depression, and fatigue.

In nonphysiological terms, Liver energy's promotion of the energy of the Heart has ramifications for:

- **Psychology:** Where anger is transformed into creativity or creative impulses are externalized as opposed to suppressed, it invariably benefits society and interpersonal relations.
- **Evolutionary theory:** The survival of the fittest principle can be expressed in generating terms. Unfettered imagination confers inadequate reproductive or metabolic advantage to any living thing. The Liver's imaginative powers morph into a motivating force that the Heart provides so that the internal challenges of environmental surroundings can be met. Evolutionary value accrues when competion with rivals and predators for food sources prompts the creative imagination to pursue strategies and tactics that are effective, viable, and synchronous with the habitat. Somehow, too, ingenius Liver creativity conjures anatomical structures such as the inimicable human eye.

(Mnenomic device: Wood can burn; in other words, catch Fire.)

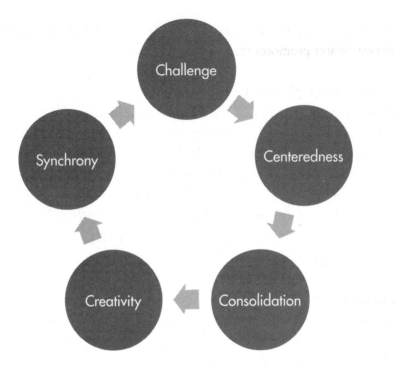

Cyclical progression through the positive poles
of the sense dimensions

FIVE STAGES OF HUMAN DEVELOPMENT

When arrayed cyclically in accordance with the TCM's Five Phases, the five sense dimensions offer a developmental model recalling Abraham Maslow's non-cyclically arrayed hierarchy of needs:

1. Physiological needs
2. Safety and security
3. Love and belonging
4. Esteem
5. Self-actualization

In our version of the generating cycle, successful resolution of a dimension's core issue provides impetus for (or sends chi toward) the challenge that resides within a succeeding dimension. Resolution of core issues embedded within the totality of the five sense dimensions not only assures a state of self-replenishing, energetic balance that denotes optimal mental, spiritual, emotional, and physical health but also provides impetus for a successful passage through the five stages of man.

- **Infancy and childhood.** When synchrony triumphs over isolation within the sense dimension of Touch, a realm of love is established under whose influence similar entities, once aligned and united of purpose, oscillate at a common wavelength and harmonize at increasingly high frequencies. Formerly separate though similar entities that so unite become a communication network capable of evolving emergent properties. Evolution of this sort includes transmutation of generic mast cells into the tissue of a specific organ and, in developmental terms, a separate individual's transformation into a social being. Ability to belong to and function as something greater than oneself is established during infancy if not sooner. Developmental entrenchment of synchrony sets the stage for:
- **Adolescence.** When challenge triumphs over anxiety within the sense dimension of Taste, a level of confidence sufficient to undertake tasks outside of a normal comfort level is established. This confidence, a desire for growth and challenge, sets the stage for:
- **Adulthood.** When centeredness triumphs over disorientation within the sense dimension of Smell, a relaxed state of acceptance with respect to what one has accomplished and where one is headed with regard to family and work is established. This state of optimal orientation sets the stage for:
- **Middle age.** When consolidation triumphs over entropy within the sense dimension of Hearing, concern shifts away from oneself and in the direction of one's legacy. The guarantors and the repository of what one has accomplished in one's life are, in fact, one's children. When our offspring and the community to which a family belongs are on a solid basis, our posterity is secured. This sets the stage for:
- **Old age.** When creativity triumphs over chaos within the sense dimension of Sight, a great freedom descends. With one's responsibilities to career, family, and society at last fulfilled, one stands

liberated from frustration and anger. One owes no obligation other than to indulge one's personal creativity, or as Maslow would put it, to self-actualize. Insofar as indulgence in one's personal creativity can eventuate in isolation, the stage is set for reentry with regard to synchrony and the concerns of infancy and childood.

TONIFICATION OF THE MOTHER, IMMERSION IN CONSOLIDATION

Failure to resolve a sense dimensional conundrum can also be expressed in terms of TCM's mother-son rule, where the strong side of a thematic axis is "deficient." An acupuncture adage within the Wuxing's Five Phases says that when a particular phase is deficient (a situation covering numerous instances of relatively low-level pathology), the treatment principle involves "tonifying" the mother. Although this directive refers specifically to stimulation of acupuncture points able to energize a phase located immediately prior to the one experiencing disruption, the following examples describe scenarios in which the effect can be accomplished by non-acupuncture means.

Resolving Problematic Synchrony

Although the "frozen" world of autistic individuals manifests an extreme state of isolation, numerous autistics are also savants, possessors of genius level ability in music, art, or mathematics. Diagnosible as blockage within the sense dimension of Touch, autism is to some extent amenable to tonification of the mother, meaning immersion within creativity, the positive pole of the immediately preceding energetic phase. Insofar as it constitutes their chief means of achieving synchrony, meaning connectedness and bonds of appreciation with neighboring individuals, autistic individuals must be helped to find, explore, and express their innate creativity. Autism spectrum disorders (ASD) present myriad challenges to the practitioner and are generally more complex than the current analysis presents. For an in-depth, homeopathic consideration of ASD see my book *Autism Reversal Toolbox: Strategies, Remedies, Resources.*

Resolving Problematic Challenge

Our interview of an excessively anxious individual leads us to diagnose a blockage related to the sense dimension of Taste, in which a history of either unreasonable parental demands (excessive challenge) or overprotectiveness (inadequate challenge) has been found to exist. Remediation is achieved by immersing this individual in synchrony, the positive pole of the immediately preceding energetic phase. The person is thus bathed in meaningful love until an embracing sense of security is regained. Whether accomplished by means of counseling, access to spiritual resources, heightened support from family and friends, homeopathy, or acupuncture, tonification of the mother energizes and prepares the individual to reengage the rigors of the anxiety-versus-challenge conundrum.

Resolving Problematic Centeredness

An interview of a functionally depressed individual reveals that the individual is mired in grief, overcome by the loss of a close personal relationship. Insofar as he is disoriented with regard to time, stuck in the past and unable to perceive the dynamism inherent in a present moment, a blockage related to the sense dimension of Smell is diagnosed. Remediation is effected by means of distracting and engaging him with an enjoyable project. Tonification of the mother, meaning immersion in challenge, the positive pole of the immediately preceding energetic phase, energizes and prepares him to reengage the rigors of the disorientation-versus-centeredness conundrum.

Resolving Problematic Consolidation

Our interview with a man maintaining that his life has fallen apart reveals a state of despair. He feels his career has been pointless, and that he is not valued within his family for anything other than his ability to put food on the table. The man's age and state of entropy direct us to diagnose a blockage within the sense dimension of Hearing. Remediation is effected by means of teaching this individual to meditate. Tonification of the mother, meaning immersion in centeredness, the positive pole of the immediately preceding energetic phase, reorients him to the original context out of which his choice of career and spouse emerged. The relaxed centeredness of the meditative state energizes and prepares him to reengage the rigors of the entropy-versus-consolidation conundrum.

Resolving Problematic Creativity

A consult with a workaholic woman complaining of headache and fatigue brings to light an immense reservoir of anger, frustration, and resentment that she harbors toward her coworkers, as well as her husband. The interview also reveals that her anger originates in a long-standing pattern of unresolved conflict with her now aged parents, whom she has never managed to please. The woman's chaotic relationships, the fact that her workplace and family expectations express hidden emotional needs, and her inability to address her problems creatively directs us to diagnose a blockage within the sense dimension of Sight.

By whatever means it can be achieved (and assuming the strategy is workable), remediation is effected by tonification of the mother, meaning immersion in consolidation, the positive pole of the immediately preceding energetic phase. Priorities are reordered such that energy withdrawn from career is redirected toward quality time spent with parents and husband. Once the woman's status within her immediate family and family of origin is thus consolidated, she is prepared to reengage with the rigors of the chaos-versus-creativity conundrum (when a reordering of her career goals is likely to occur).

JOURNEY'S END

Safely through the Strait

Onward we sail, Charybdis
amidst her whirlpool
of chronic illness to the left
To the right cancerous Scylla
stewing in her deceits, grievances
rage and tormented yearnings

At the horizon
old age beckons
the safe harbor
of a life fulfilled.

Did I live synchronously with nature and with
    others?
Were anxieties surmounted, the challenges of
    my life engaged?
Despite strictures of time and place, did I
    breathe freely?
Was a legacy for my descendants secured?
Has the insurrection of my birth been fruitful?

Modeling Explanations

Are the interpretations of Fire and Earth in conflict with one another? Which of the phases best explains Sulphur? The one according with my sketchbook notion, the Fire phase? Or, vis-a-vis psora, the Earth phase according with the miasm-based model? Are the interpretations of Fire and Earth in conflict with one another? A foray into philosophy can help.

Common sense says that explanations should show us a cause and its effect. Yet the how or why questions to which we are limited fail to produce cause-and-effect answers. The how of something elicits a description, such as when my doctor seeks to explain my soft tissue pain by labeling it "fibromyalgia," when this provides no more than a Latin translation of already described symptoms. Or in a sequence of events that philosophers term "phenomena": My nose bled because you punched it. Here is a seemingly causal relationship. Yet strictly speaking two separate phenomena, a punch and my bleeding nose, are juxtaposed. Rather than, "This made that happen," it is more accurate to say, "Such and such happened, followed by such and such happening." Prosecuting attorneys will disagree but (to varying extents) all causality has to be considered circumstantial.

The answer to a why question wants to bridge divergent events. This requires a conjecture. To be predictive the conjecture must be tested. The testing can be operational, as in attending to new evidence at hand, or conceptual, meaning reliant on coherence. Upon passing such tests the conjecture becomes theory. Then, so that a theory's applicability can expand, a working model of the theory's possibilities is developed. Explanatory models engender much tinkering. A model tends to sprout corollaries that bolster, stretch, or restrict the theory's applicability. Over time a model's acceptance and elaboration allow it to provide support and context for derivative theories from which alternative explanatory models develop. When the selfsame question is visited by divergent theories whose dissimilar premises are defensible, their respective models need not stand in contradiction to one another. Hence the remedy Sulphur, on the one hand viewed as overindulgence of the sketchpad of joy, and the remedy Sulphur viewed as the king of psora on the other, are not incompatible.

Resources for Other Existential Perspectives on Homeopathy

MICHAL YAKIR

Michal Yakir, author of *Wondrous Order: Systematic Table of Homeopathic Plant Remedies,* is an Israeli botanist, gardener, homeopath, researcher, and educator. She has developed a remarkable system that organizes the plant kingdom according to an accessible, tabular set of coordinates. The system enables prediction of common characteristics among plant families and their members. The intersection of row and column pegs denotes the profile of a patient, featuring specific existential issues, psychological traits, and physical pathologies.

The table of plants maps the parallel between plant group evolution (rooted in Arthur Cronquist's botanic taxonomy) and the developmental journey of mankind and cosmic forces. Woven into the wondrous fabric of the plant kingdom are insights drawn from psychology that include interplay between feminine and masculine archetypes, philosophy, and Kabbala. While expanding homeopathy's existential relevance, Yakir's work has enriched homeopathic materia medica.

JAN SCHOLTEN

Homeopaths need no introduction to Dutch physician Jan Scholten, renowned author of seminal texts including *Homeopathy and the Elements, Homeopathy and Minerals, Secret Lanthanides,* and others.

The elements of the periodic table are building blocks of the universe. How wonderful it is that not only does each element have a distinct personality (usually aligned with the history, mythic or otherwise, of the personage for whom the element has been named), but its rows and columns represent existential and developmental life themes.

The columns of the periodic table comprise eighteen stages in a process of development charting a rise, culmination, and decline within existential categories pertaining to being, identity, work, creativity, power, and magus (deep spiritual meaning). Scholten's work is both philosophically enthralling and immensely practical, since it elucidates known remedies and important new ones.

PETER TUMMINELLO

The Australian homeopath is also a gemologist and author of *Twelve Jewels: Gems in Homeopathy* and *Psyche and Structure: Crystals and Minerals in Homeopathy.*

In a review of *Psyche and Structure* Misha Norland, a founding member of the Society of Homeopaths, wrote, "Peter Tumminello has uncovered universal morphologies, crystal geometries that underlie the world of manifestation. He then links these with pathology and the subtle structures of the human psyche."

My own experience with gemstone and crystal remedies shows that they are existentially profound. I will let Peter Tumminello explain the various reasons:

- They instruct us to resolve the conflict between instinctual and enlightened attitudes. "Commonly manifest in the gems is a battle between the lower aspects of self, the more animal, instinctual or inert aspects of human behavior, and the aspects that enhance an intelligent response to our world of experiences. The lower aspects are highlighted in the animal images—violence, abuse, and want of feeling that pervade the gems as a group. The enlightened attitudes are highlighted by the positivity, big picture consciousness, and awareness/understanding that the gems evoke.

"There is a feeling that these opposites need to be reconciled and there is a strong conscious tension between them that is often expressed as the desire for connection, whether with self or others. This desire for connection is a search for the solution to the tensions between these natural worldly and emancipated thoughts. In Diamond, for example, it is the desire to connect with perfection versus the stress of doing so, without understanding that it involves a process and the need for loving oneself. In Sapphire, the tension is between survival instincts and the maintenance of one's caring humanity."

- They instruct us about the elemental interaction of yin and yang. "Many crystals are the result of the resolution of powerful elemental forces that appear irreconcilable. Yin and yang, light and dark, good and evil, male and female, life and death, fire and water, love and hate, confusion and order are all recurrent themes of the gems. There is a distinct current of consciousness grappling with the larger issues related to these forces, not unlike the forces of nature that are aligned to produce these marvelous substances. For example, fundamental male/female issues are largely dealt with in Emerald and Ruby, love and hate in Amethyst, and life and death in Diamond."

- They bring crystalized belief systems into the light. "When talking to a gem cutter about a beautiful red zircon I had cut, we were admiring its magical beauty and he commented, 'And it will last you only 400,000 years!' Gems are old, really old, and are indicated for the oldest and most solidified of belief systems. Those beliefs about race, religion, sexuality, and the nature of human existence are particularly at stake. Sapphire, Black opal, and Lapis are the outstanding remedies for gaining a new perspective but many of the gems generate a powerful change in consciousness and perspective. Have you ever heard of the phrase, 'He has got rocks in his head?'"[1]

Notes

PREFACE

1. App, trans., ed., *Master Yunmen,* 177, 185.

CONTEXTUALIZING THE LAW OF SIMILARS

1. Bell and Schwartz, "Adaptive Network Nanomedicine," 685–708.
2. Montagnier et al., "Electromagnetic Signals Are Produced by Aqueous Nanostructures."

PSYCHIC EXCAVATION

1. Homer, *The Odyssey,* book 11, line 567.
2. Tumminello, *Twelve Jewels,* 13–53.
3. Scholten, *Homeopathy and the Elements,* 719–24.
4. Melville, *Bartleby, the Scrivener,* paragraph 21.
5. Scholten, *Homeopathy and the Elements,* 793–97.
6. Scholten, *Homeopathy and the Elements*, 350–53.
7. Scholten, *Homeopathy and the Elements,* 492–95.
8. Scholten, *Homeopathy and the Elements,* 653–58.
9. Scholten, *Homeopathy and the Elements,* 653–56.

CHAPTER 1. AM I ALONE IN LIFE OR DO I ACT IN SYNCHRONY WITH NATURE AND WITH OTHERS?

1. Hertenstein et al., "Communication of Emotion via Touch."
2. Gick and Derrick, "Aero-tactile Integration in Speech Perception," 502–4.
3. Human Microbiome Project Consortium, "Structure, Function, and Diversity," 207–14.
4. Ohm, "Shifting the Paradigm."

5. World Population Review website, "Mumbai Population 2023," accessed January 14, 2023.

6. Kay Johnson, "Census."

7. Heudens-Mast and Divine, *Foundation of the Chronic Miasms*.

8. *Encyclopedia Britannica*, "Tuberculosis: Pathology," Britannica (online), last updated January 5, 2023.

9. Krishnan, *Phantom Plague*, 9–23.

10. Strogatz, *Sync*, 11–39.

11. Donne, *Devotions upon Emergent Occasions*, meditation xvii.

12. Hering, "Guiding Symptoms of Our Materia Medica."

CHAPTER 2. *IS MY PRESENCE IN THE WORLD SUSTAINABLE?*

1. App, trans., ed., *Master Yunmen*, 102.

2. Kantor, "Cyclical Remedy Complexes," 202–7.

3. Kafka, *Selected Short Stories*, 3–18.

4. Fraser, *Birds*, 5.

5. Proving conducted by Misha Norland at the School of Homeopathy in 1998, edited and collated by Peter Fraser. Available on the School of Homeopathy website; see under The School/Provings/Peregrine Falcon.

6. Sankaran, *Substance of Homeopathy*, 169–70.

7. Sankaran, *Spirit of Homeopathy*, 298.

CHAPTER 3. *AM I ORIENTED IN SPACE AND TIME?*

1. Dallek, *Unfinished Life*, 102.

2. Dallek, *Unfinished Life*, 123.

3. National Library of Medicine website, "Urethritis," last updated December 1, 2022.

4. Dallek, *Unfinished Life*, 195, 212.

5. Hompath website, "Sycotic Miasm—Understanding the Miasmatic Symptoms," August 27, 2019; originating from Speight, *Study Course in Homeopathy*.

6. Kantor, *Interpreting Chronic Illness*, 99.

7. Yakir, *Wondrous Order*, 99.

8. Yakir, *Wondrous Order*, 370.

9. Yakir, *Wondrous Order*, 370–71.

10. Kreiner, *The Wandering Mind*, 1–19.

11. Szalai, "Think Screens Stole Our Attention?"

12. Cep, "Eat, Pray, Concentrate," 56–57.

13. Hering, "Guiding Symptoms of Our Materia Medica."

14. Livy, *Early History of Rome,* book 1, chapter 9.

15. Scholten, *Secret Lanthanides,* 195.

16. Yakir, *Wondrous Order,* 99.

17. Evans, *Meditative Provings,* vol. 1, 242.

18. Stephen Johnson and Winters, *Mistletoe and the Emerging Future.*

19. Paulina Medical Clinic, "New Uses for Mistletoe–Viscum Album 25X."

20. Tong et al., "p53 Frameshift Mutations," 1522–33.

21. Chang et al., "High Frequency of Frameshift Mutation," 195–204.

22. Ramakrishnan, *My Homeopathic Method,* 15–16, 183–89. This elaborates on Ramakrishnan's earlier exposition on plussing provided in his first book, *A Homeopathic Approach to Cancer,* 183–88.

CHAPTER 4. CAN THE BOUNDARY
BETWEEN LIFE AND DEATH BE ABIDED?

1. University of Michigan, "Syphilis Topic Overview."

2. Abram, *Spell of the Sensuous,* 128–30.

3. Scholten, *Homeopathy and the Elements,* 592.

4. Vermeulen, *Prisma,* 910.

5. Soniak, "Why Is a Fake Doctor Called a Quack?"

CHAPTER 5. WILL THE INSURRECTION
OF MY BIRTH PROVE FRUITFUL?

1. De Gelder et al., "Intact Navigational Skills."

2. American Academy of Ophthalmology EyeWiki website, "Visual Snow," last updated March 13, 2023.

3. Klein, *Miasms and Nosodes,* 407–37.

APPENDIX B. RESOURCES FOR
OTHER EXISTENTIAL PERSPECTIVES ON HOMEOPATHY

1. Tumminello, "Introduction to the Gem Family."

Bibliography

Abram, David. *The Spell of the Sensuous: Perception and Language in a More-than-Human World*. New York: Vintage Books, 1997.

Anderson, Paul Thomas. *There Will Be Blood*. Prod. Ghoulardi Film Company, 2007.

App, Urs, trans., ed. *Master Yunmen: From the Record of the Chan Master "Gate of the Clouds."* Tokyo: Kodansha International, 1994.

Beckett, Samuel. *Waiting for Godot*. New York: Grove Press, 2011.

Bell, Iris R., and Gary E. Schwartz. "Adaptive Network Nanomedicine: An Integrated Model for Homeopathic Medicine." *Frontiers in Bioscience* 5, no. 2 (2013): 685–708.

Binswanger, Ludwig. *Being in the World: Selected Papers of Ludwig Binswanger*. Jacob Needleman, trans. New York: Harper & Row, 1967.

Buber, Martin. *I and Thou*. Eastford, Conn.: Martino Publishing, 2010.

Camus, Albert. *The Myth of Sisyphus and Other Essays*. Justin O'Brien, trans. 2nd ed., New York: Alfred K. Knopf, 1969.

Cep, Casey. "Eat, Pray, Concentrate: What Monks Can Teach Us about Paying Attention." *New Yorker,* January 30, 2023: 56–57.

Chang, Mae Yin, Inn-Wen Chong, Fang-Ming Chen, Jaw-Yuan Wang, Yian-Lu Cheng, Yu-Jen Cheng, Chau Chyun Sheu, Sung-hu Hung, Ming-Chen Yang, and Shiu-Ru Lin. "High Frequency of Frameshift Mutation on p53 Gene in Taiwanese with Non-small Cell Lung Cancer." Presented by *Cancer Letter* on PubMed website. Accessed January 28, 2023: 195–204.

Cicchetti, Jane. *Dreams, Symbols, and Homeopathy: Archetypal Dimensions of Healing*. Berkeley: North Atlantic, 2003.

Dallek, Robert. *An Unfinished Life: John F. Kennedy 1917–1963*. Boston: Little, Brown, 2003.

De Gelder, Beatrice, Marco Tamietto, Geert van Boxtel, Rainer Goebel, Arash Sahraie, Jan van den Stock, Bernard M. C. Stienen, Lawrence Weiskrantz, and Alan Pegna. "Intact Navigational Skills after Bilateral Loss of Striate

Cortex." Presented by *Current Biology* on PubMed website. Accessed January 26, 2023: R1128–29.

Donne, John. *Devotions upon Emergent Occasions.* Oxford, U.K.: Oxford University Press, 1987.

Evans, Madeline. *Meditative Provings,* vol. 1. Middlesex, U.K.: The Rose Press, 2000.

Frankl, Viktor. *Man's Search for Meaning.* Boston: Beacon Press, 2006.

Fraser, Peter. *Birds: Seeking the Freedom of the Sky.* Ongar, U.K.: Good News Press, 2009.

Freud Sigmund. *Civilization and Its Discontents.* New York: W. W. Norton, 2010.

Gick, Brian, and Donald Derrick. "Aero-tactile Integration in Speech Perception." *Nature* online journal (2009). Accessed January 29, 2023: 502–4.

Heidegger, Martin. *Basic Writings: From* Being and Time *(1927) to the* Task of Thinking *(1964).* David F. Krell, ed. San Francisco: HarperCollins, 1993.

Hering, Constantine. "The Guiding Symptoms of Our Materia Medica." Presented by Médi-T on Homéopathe International Website. Accessed February 1, 2023.

Hertenstein, Matthew J., Rachel Holmes, Margaret McCullough, and Dacher Keltner. "The Communication of Emotion via Touch." *Emotion* (August 9, 2009): 566–73.

Heudens-Mast, Henny, and Louise Divine. *The Foundation of the Chronic Miasms in the Practice of Homeopathy.* Deland, Fla.: Similia Press. 2005.

Homer. *The Odyssey.* A. T. Murray, PhD, ed. Cambridge, Mass.: Harvard University Press, 1919.

Human Microbiome Project Consortium. "Structure, Function and Diversity of the Healthy Human Microbiome." *Nature* website (June 13, 2012). Accessed February 1, 2023: 207–14.

Johnson, Kay. "Census: 1 in 6 India City Residents Lives in Slums." *San Diego Union-Tribune* online, March 22, 2013.

Johnson, Stephen, and Nasha Winters. *Mistletoe and the Emerging Future of Integrative Oncology.* Portal Books digital publishing, 2021.

Kafka, Franz. *Selected Short Stories.* With an introduction by Philip Rahv. New York: Modern Library, n.d.

Kantor, Jerry. *Autism Reversal Toolbox, Strategies, Remedies, Resources.* Rev. ed. Haarlem, Netherlands: Emryss, 2022.

———. "Cyclical Remedy Complexes: Their Origin within Traditional Chinese Medicine and Relevance for Miasmatic Theory." Homeopathic Links, Thieme Medical and Scientific Publishers (2017): 202–207.

———. *Interpreting Chronic Illness, the Convergence of Traditional Chinese Medicine, Homeopathy and Biomedicine.* Needham, Mass.: Right Whale Press, 2012.

Kierkegaard, Soren. *Fear and Trembling.* New York: Penguin Classics, 1986.

Klein, Louis. *Miasms and Nosodes: Origins of Disease.* Kandern, Germany: Narayana Verlag, 2009: 407–37.

Kreiner, Jamie. *The Wandering Mind: What Medieval Monks Tell Us About Distraction.* New York: Liveright, 2023.

Krishnan, Vidya. *The Phantom Plague: How Tuberculosis Shaped History.* New York: *Public Affairs,* 2022.

Livy, Titus. *The Early History of Rome, Books I–V.* New York: Penguin Classics, 2002.

May, Rollo. *Man's Search for Himself.* New York: W. W. Norton, 2009.

Melville, Herman. *Bartleby, the Scrivener: A Story of Wall Street* (Brooklyn, N.Y.: Melville House Books, 2004).

Milton, John. *Paradise Lost.* London: Penguin Classics, 2009.

Montagnier, Luc, Jamal Aissa, Stéphane Ferris, Jean-Luc Montagnier, and Claude Lavallee. "Electromagnetic Signals Are Produced by Aqueous Nanostructures Derived from Bacterial DNA Sequences." Heidelberg, Germany: *Interdisciplinary Sciences.*(2009). Presented by PubMed website. Accessed February 1, 2023: 81–90.

Nietzsche, Friedrich. *Will to Power.* London: Penguin Classics, 2017.

Ohm, Jeanne. "Shifting the Paradigm: Insight into the Germ Theory–Trusting the Process." Charlottesville Family Chiropractic website (May 10, 2018). Accessed April 16, 2022.

Paulina Medical Clinic. "New Uses for Mistletoe–Viscum Album 25X." Paulina Medical Clinic website. Accessed April 16, 2022.

Ramakrishnan, A. U. *A Homeopathic Approach to Cancer.* St. Louis: Quality Medical Publishing, 2001.

———. *My Homeopathic Method.* Kandern, Germany: Narayana Verlag, 2016.

Sankaran, Rajan. *The Spirit of Homeopathy.* Mumbai: Homeopathic Medical Publishers, 2008.

———.*The Substance of Homeopathy.* Mumbai: Homeopathic Medical Publishers, 1999.

Sartre, Jean-Paul. *Being and Nothingness*. 2nd ed. Abingdon, Oxfordshire, U.K.: Routledge, 2003.

Scholten, Jan. *Homeopathy and Minerals*. Berkeley, Calif.: Homeopathic Educational Services, 2006.

———. *Homeopathy and the Elements*. Translated by Marriette Honig. Berkeley, Calif.: Homeopathic Educational Services, 2007.

———. *Secret Lanthanides*. Utrecht, Netherlands: Stichting Alonnissos, 2005.

———. *Wonderful Plants*. Utrecht, Netherlands: Stichting Alonissos, 2013.

Sheldrake, Rupert. *Morphic Resonance: The Nature of Formative Causation*. Rochester, Vt.: Park Street Press, 2009.

Soniak, Matt. "Why Is a Fake Doctor Called a Quack?" Mental Floss website, January 23, 2013.

Speight, Phyllis. *Study Course in Homeopathy*. Essex, U.K.: C. W. Daniel Company, Ltd., 1980.

Strogatz, Steven. *Sync: The Emerging Science of Spontaneous Order*. New York: Hachette, 2003.

Szalai, Jennifer. "Think Screens Stole Our Attention? Medieval Monks Were Distracted Too." *New York Times Book Review,* January 9, 2023.

Tong, David R., Wen Zhou, Chen Katz, Kausik Regunath, Divya Venkatesh, Chinyere Ihuegbu, James J. Manfredi, Oleg Laptenko, and Carol Prives. "p53 Frameshift Mutations Couple Loss-of-Function with Unique Neomorphic Activities." *Molecular Cancer Research* 19, no. 9 (September 2021). Presented by AACR Journals website: 1522–33.

Tumminello, Peter. "Introduction to the Gem Family." *Interhomeopathy International Homeopathic Internet Journal,* February 2011.

———. *Psyche and Structure*. Kandern, Germany: Narayana Verlag, 2017.

———. *Twelve Jewels*. Marrickville, Australia: Southwood Press, 2005.

University of Michigan *Healthwise* Staff. "Syphilis Topic Overview." Accessed February 26, 2020.

Vermeulen, Frans. *Prisma: The Arcana of Materia Medica Illuminated*. Haarlem, Netherlands: Emryss, 2002.

Yakir, Michal. *Wondrous Order: Systematic Table of Homeopathic Plant Remedies*. Kandern, Germany: Narayana Verlag, 2017.

Yalom, Irvin D. *Staring at the Sun: Overcoming the Terror of Death*. San Francisco: Jossey-Bass, 2009.

Yasgur, Jay. *Yasgur's Homeopathic Dictionary and Holistic Health Reference*. 6th ed. Terre Haute, Ind.: Van Hoy, 2021.

Index

Page numbers in *italics* refer to illustrations.